Natural Health Products Compendium

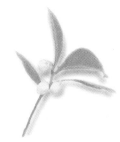

**The Guide to Nutritional Supplements,
Herbs, Homeopathics
and Other Natural Products**

Natural Health
Products
Compendium

Alive Research Group

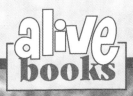

Published by

Natural Life Publishing, Inc.
250 – H – Street #8110-357
Blaine, WA
USA 98230
(800) 663-6580
(800) 661-0303

Natural Life Publishing, Inc.
PO Box 80055
Burnaby, BC
Canada V5H 3X1
(604) 435-1919 (800) 663-6513
Fax 800-663-6597

If you intend to use the information presented in this book without the approval of a
health professional, you are prescribing for yourself, which is your right, but the publisher
assumes no responsibility.
This book is intended only as an informative guide for those wishing to know more about
vitamins, minerals, supplements and herbs.
The information in this book is general and is offered with no guarantees on the part of
the publisher of alive books.
The inclusion of a manufacturer's product listing in the **Natural Health Products
Compendium** does not imply that the editors endorse or recommend these products as
being clinically superior to similar products of any other firm.
Users are advised that the information provided in the **Natural Health Products
Compendium** is not exhaustive, other sources may contain additional information.

Printing: January 1998

Canadian Cataloguing in Publication Data

Natural Health Products Compendium

ISBN 0-920470-72-6
 1. Medicine, Popular–Directories. 2. Dietary Supplements–Directories. 3. Nutrition–Directories.
4. Herbs–Directories. 5. Homeopathy–Directories.
RC81.N37 1998   616.02'4   C97-910924-8

Printed and bound in Canada

A Message from
Siegfried Gursche, Publisher

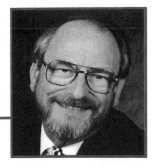

Dear Reader,

Never before in history have so many people wanted to learn about the principles of natural health and the benefits of choosing natural health products. This compendium is designed as a resource to provide current, concise information about nutritional supplements, herbs, homeopathic remedies, etc. It is designed for consumers and health stores, as well as medical doctors, naturopaths, and other health professionals.

As a health enthusiast and natural health products consumer, you must have often wanted to obtain more information about a nutritional supplement, a homeopathic remedy or herbal preparation. Finally, the **Natural Health Products Compendium** provides the ideal way to get critical information pertaining to natural health products—the ingredients, directions for use, contra-indications, possible side-effects and much more.

With this first edition of the **Natural Health Products Compendium**, we have created a quick reference guide to over 750 products. **alive** Books will revise, update, and expand this guide at regular intervals. We are dedicated to providing you with the natural health care information you need to make the best choices for yourself, your family or your clients.

Yours in good health,

Siegfried Gursche, MH
Publisher

Table of Contents

*All products are listed in alphabetical order.

Table of Symbols

🏠	Manufacturer	💧	Liquid
	Distributor	🥄	Powder
	Ingredients		Tablet
	Dosage		Tincture
	Product Packaging		Tonic or Syrup
	Information		Side Effects
	Capsule		Contra-Indications
	Cream application		Visual Identification
	Herbal Tea		

Product
Listings

Section I

Products are listed alphabetically. Immediately following the product name the manufacturer is listed. *For complete address information see Section II- Manufacturer and Distributor Listing.* Each entry consists of product ingredients, dosage, side-effects, contra-indications, product packaging, additional information and visual identification.

100% Pure Aloe Vera Gel
Certified Organic

🏠 **Aubrey Organics®**

⚗️ Contains: Organic Aloe vera gel (extract from inside leaf), Aloe vera oil, Citrus seed extract with Vitamins A, C and E as preservatives.

✋ Shake well, apply to affected area.

📦 Available in 4 oz.

ℹ️ External use only. Vegan.

🧴 Gel.

Acidophilus & Bifidus
5 Billion Active Cells

🏠 **Natural Factors® Nutritional Products Ltd.**

⚗️ Each capsule contains: 5 billion active cells of the following specially cultured strains of probiotics (at time of manufacture): L. rhamnosus 80% 4.00 billion, L. acidophilus 10% 0.50 billion, B. bifidum 10% 0.50 billion. These micro-organisms are in a base of powdered Goat's milk. Magnesium stearate (used as a lubricant), Pectin, Ascorbic acid in a gelatin capsule.

✋ Take 3 capsules daily at mealtime.

📦 Available in 90 and 180 capsules.

ℹ️ Internal use. At time of manufacture guaranteed minimum 5 billion active cells per capsule.

💊 Capsule.

📷 Visual.

Acidophilus & Bifidus
Double Strength

🏠 **Natural Factors® Nutritional Products Ltd.**

⚗️ Each capsule contains: 10 billion active cells of the following specially cultured strains of probiotics: L. rhamnosus 80% 8.00 billion, L. acidophilus 10% 1.00 billion, B. bifidum 10% 1.00 billion. Magnesium stearate (used as a lubricant), pectin, ascorbic acid in a gelatin capsule.

✋ Take 3 capsules daily at mealtime.

📦 Available in 90 and 180 capsules.

ℹ️ Internal use. Contains no artificial preservatives, color, corn, gluten, soya, starch, sweeteners or yeast. These micro-organisms are in a base of powdered Goat's milk. At time of manufacture guaranteed minimum 10 billion active cells per capsule.

💊 Capsule.

📷 Visual.

Acidophilus Powder
Children's Formula

🏠 **Natural Factors® Nutritional Products Ltd.**

⚗️ Each 1/4 tsp. (1g) contains: 2 billion active cells of the following specially cultured strains of probiotics. L. rhamnosus 65% 1.30 billion, B. infants 20% 0.40 billion, S. thermophilus 9.9% 0.19 billion, L. acidophilus 5% 0.10 billion, L. delbrueckii subsp. bulgaricus 0.1% 0.01 billion to maintain healthful balance. These micro-organisms are in a base of powdered Malto-dextrin, Strawberry flavor, and Ascorbic acid.

✋ Take 1/4 tsp. at mealtime. Mix in juices, protein drinks or sprinkle on cereal or fruit.

📦 Available in 50 g.

ℹ️ Internal use. Contains no artificial preservatives, color, corn, dairy, soya, starch or yeast. At time of manufacture guaranteed minimum 2 billion active cells per gram.

🥄 Powder.

📷 Visual.

Acne Gel
Homeopathic Cream

🏠 **A. Nelson & Company Ltd.**

⚗️ Contains: Extracts of organically grown Hypericum perforatum 1x 2.5%, Calendula officinalis 1x 2.5%, Arnica montana 1x 2.5%, Sulfur 6x 1.5%, and Tea tree oil, in a water-soluble gel base.

✋ Cleanse area thoroughly and apply to pimples and blemishes.

📦 27 g tube.

External use. Organic. Not tested on animals.

Gel.

Avoid contact with eyes. If symptoms persist, consult a physician.

Aconite
Homeopathic Remedy

A. Nelson & Company Ltd.

Each pillule contains: Aconitum napellus 6c.

Take 2 pillules every 2 hours for the first 6 doses, then 4 times daily for up to 5 days. Pillules should be sucked or chewed and taken between meals.

84 pillules/globules per bottle.

Internal use.

Pillule/globule.

Actea Rac.
Homeopathic Remedy

A. Nelson & Company Ltd.

Each pillule contains: Actea racemosa 6c.

Take 2 pillules every 2 hours for the first 6 doses, then 4 times daily for up to 5 days. Pillules should be sucked or chewed and taken between meals.

84 pillules/globules per bottle.

Internal use.

Pillule/globule.

Activated Charcoal
260 mg

Nature's Herbs®

Each 260 mg capsule contains: USP Grade Activated charcoal.

Take 2 capsules with each meal. Repeat in one hour if needed; not to exceed 16 capsules per day.

100 capsules.

Internal use. Preservative-free.

Capsule.

Advanced Glucosamine Sulfate
Complex with Turmeric

Quest Vitamins

Each capsule contains: Glucosamine sulfate (sodium free) 200 mg, N-Acetyl glucosamine 200 mg, Turmeric (95% curcuminoids) 100 mg, Magnesium stearate (vegetable source). Capsule shell: Gelatin, Water.

Take 2 to 4 capsules daily or as directed by a health professional.

Available in 90 capsules.

Internal use. Contains no artificial preservatives, colors, flavors or added sugar, starch, milk products wheat or yeast. Sodium free.

Capsule.

Agrimony
Bach Flower Remedy

Bach Flower Remedies® Ltd.

Contains: Agrimonia eupatoria 5x in 27% grape alcohol solution.

Take 2 drops under the tongue 4 times daily or 2 drops in a small glass of spring water and sip at intervals.

10 ml with dropper.

Internal use.

Liquid.

Alfalfa Leaf

Nature's Herbs®

Each 374 mg capsule contains: Certified organically grown Alfalfa leaf.

Take 3-4 capsules 3 times daily with a large glass of water.

Available in 100 capsules.

Internal use. Preservative-free.

Capsule.

Alkyrol® Shark Liver Oil

Scandinavian Natural Health & Beauty Products, Inc.

Contains: Shark liver oil, standardized to contain 20% alkylglycerols. Capsule ingredients: Gelatine and Glycerine.

For prevention: take 250 mg 2-3 times daily. For therapeutic effect: take 500 mg 3 times daily.

Available in blister packs of 60 and 120 capsules of 250 mg and 120 capsules of 500 mg.

Internal use. Soft gel capsules containing extensively purified oil from the liver of cold-water sharks (contains no Vitamin A or D).

Capsule.

ALLER-AWAY®

Homeopathic Complex

A. Nelson & Company Ltd.

Each tablet contains: Allium cepa 6c, Euphrasia officinalis 6c, Sabadilla officinarum 6c.

Suck or chew 2 tablets every hour for 6 doses (12 tablets). Then 2 tablets 3 times daily until symptoms subside.

72 tablets in blister packs.

Internal use.

Tablet.

Aller-Ease Formula

Natural Factors® Nutritional Products Ltd.

Each capsule contains: Brigham tea extract (Ephedra nevadensis) 50 mg, Licorice

extract (12% Glycyrrhizin) (Glycyrrhiza glabra) 50 mg, Proanthoxidants™ (85% Polyphenols) 10 mg, Wild cherry bark powder (Prunus serotina) 100 mg, Quercetin 50 mg, in a gelatin capsule with rice protein.

Take 1-3 capsules daily.

Available in 90 capsules.

Internal use. Contains no artificial preservatives, color, dairy, sweeteners, starch, wheat or yeast.

Capsule.

Visual.

Aloe Seltzer™

Aloe-Vitamin C Cocktail

Nutraceutics Corporation

Each tablet contains: Vitamin C 1000 mg (L-Ascorbic acid) U.S.P., Betamannin™ 50 mg, Standardized Lypholized whole Aloe vera gel (200:1 extract) with specific polysaccharide/glycopeptide complex in a base of bicarbonate of soda and citric acid.

Dissolve 1 or 2 tablets per 2 oz. of water. Stir before drinking.

Available in Tube, box and case.

Internal use. Effervescent. Naturally sweetened & flavored.

Effervescent tablet.

Aloe Vera Gel

Nature's Herbs®

Each capsule contains: Premium concentrated Aloe vera gel 200:1 (equivalent to 5000 mg.) in a base of cold-processed soybean oil, vegetable oil and silica in a softgel shell of gelatin, glycerin and purified water.

Take 3-6 capsules daily with water. For external purposes, simply puncture the soft gel and squeeze out the contents. Use as any fresh Aloe vera gel for soothing, emollient benefits.

Available in 30 softgel capsules.

Internal and external use.

Softgel capsule.

Aloe Vera Inner Leaf

Nature's Herbs®

Each capsule contains: Premium Aloe vera inner leaf in a soothing botanical base of Arrowroot and Fennel Seed, Gelatin.

Take 2-3 capsules 2-3 times daily with a full glass of water.

100 capsules.

Internal use. Preservative-free.

Capsule.

Alpenkraft Herbal Cough Candies

🏠 **Salus-Haus**

⚗️ Contains: Herbal extracts of: Plantain, Soapwort, Thyme, Sage, Lichen, Licorice. Essential oils of: Thyme, Pine, Eucalyptus, Fennel, Peppermint. Malt extract, Mint extract, Honey, Cane sugar/glucose.

👋 Suck on lozenge as needed.

📦 Available in package of 75 g/20 lozenges.

Ⅱ Internal use. Herbal cough candies. Especially suitable for: Smokers, athletes, singers and public speakers.

Alpenkraft Herbal Cough Syrup

🏠 **Salus-Haus**

⚗️ Each tsp. contains: 2.1 g decoction and distillate from: Medicinal ingredients: Thyme herb 38.5 mg, Camomile flowers 8.5 mg, Milfoil herb 8.5 mg, Linden flowers 8.5 mg, Primrose flowers 7.5 mg, Aniseed 6.00 mg, Caraway 6.0 mg, Fennel 6.0 mg, Sundew 5.5 mg, Hops cones 4.5 mg, Knotgrass 2.75 mg, Dwarf pine extract 25.8 mg, Dwarf pine oil 3.6 mg, Aniseed oil 0.8 mg, Fennel oil 0.8 mg, Eucalyptus oil 0.4 mg, in a base of: Honey 1.875 g, Malt extract 0.200 g, Licorice extract 0.013 g.

👋 Take 1 tsp. 3-4 times daily and slowly dissolve in mouth before swallowing. School age children may use the same amount as adults.

📦 Available in 10 ml trial size, 250 ml.

Ⅱ Internal use.

💧 Cough syrup.

Aminoderm Gel

🏠 **Aubrey Organics®**

⚗️ Contains: Witch hazel, water, Amino acid complex, Vitamin A, Goa herb. Mineral-herb complex (Magnesium, Zinc, Burdock, Ivy, lemon, Sage, Saponin, Watercress) Allantoin and Camomile.

👋 Apply a small amount once or twice daily after washing.

📦 Available in 2 oz.

Ⅱ External use only. Vegan.

🧴 Gel.

Apis Mel.
Homeopathic Remedy

🏠 **A. Nelson & Company Ltd.**

⚗️ Each pillule contains: Apis mellifica 6c.

👋 Take 2 pillules every 2 hours for the first 6 doses, then 4 times daily for up to 5 days. Pillules should be sucked or chewed and taken between meals.

📦 84 pillules/globules per bottle.

Ⅱ Internal use.

⊘ Pillule/globule.

Argent. Nit.
Homeopathic Remedy

🏠 **A. Nelson & Company Ltd.**

⚗️ Each pillule contains: Argentum nitricum 6c.

👋 Take 2 pillules every 2 hours for the first 6 doses, then 4 times daily for up to 5 days. Pillules should be sucked or chewed and taken between meals.

📦 84 pillules/globules per bottle.

Ⅱ Internal use.

⊘ Pillule/globule.

Arnica
Homeopathic Remedy

🏠 **A. Nelson & Company Ltd.**

⚗️ Each pillule contains: Arnica montana 6c.

👋 Take 2 pillules every 2 hours for the first 6 doses, then 4 times daily for up to 5 days. Pillules should be sucked or chewed and taken between meals.

📦 84 pillules/globules per bottle.

Ⅱ Internal use.

⊘ Pillule/globule.

Arnica Cream

Homeopathic Cream

A. Nelson & Company Ltd.

Contains: Extract of organically grown Arnica montana 1x 9% in a base of almond oil, avocado oil and cocoa butter.

Apply gently to bruised areas.

27 g tube.

External use. Organic. Not tested on animals.

Cream.

Avoid contact with eyes. If symptoms persist, consult a physician.

Arnica Tincture

Salus-Haus

Each 10 g tincture contains: 10 g extract derived from 1 g of Arnica blossoms.

Put 5 to 10 drops onto a piece of watersoaked gauze covering the affected portion of the body.

Available in 50 ml, includes a dropper.

External use only. It is especially effective for external use as a compress for bruises, swellings, sprains and contusions; also applied to cuts and scrapes. Salus herbal tinctures are made in accordance with strictest health food principles, using natural ingredients only.

Tincture.

Application on injured skin over a long period of time may cause edematous dermatitis including vesiculation.

Allergies to Arnica may to occur in rare cases.

Arsen. alb.

Homeopathic Remedy

A. Nelson & Company Ltd.

Each pillule contains: Arsenicum album 6c.

Take 2 pillules every 2 hours for the first 6 doses, then 4 times daily for up to 5 days. Pillules should be sucked or chewed and taken between meals.

84 pillules/globules per bottle.

Internal use.

Pillule/globule.

Art-R

naka Sales Ltd.

Each capsule contains: approximately 400 mg of the following herbs: Devil's claw, Milk thistle, White willow bark, Burdock root, Dandelion root, Yucca.

Take 1 or 2 capsules 3 times daily with each meal or as directed by a professional.

Available in 150 capsules.

Internal use.

Gelatin capsules.

Not be taken if suffering from gastric ulcer.

Artesian Acres Spelt

Artesian Acres Inc.

Contains: Spelt.

Organic food. Allergy testing has confirmed that spelt is well tolerated by the wheat sensitive. Spelt is available as whole grain, flakes and flour as well as breakfast cereal, breads, mixes etc.

Arth Plus®

Nature's Herbs®

Each capsule contains: Yucca, White willow bark, Hydrangea root, Devil's claw, Alfalfa leaves, Burdock root, Black cohosh root, Sarsaparilla root, Prickly ash bark, Slippery elm bark, Cayenne, Trace minerals, Licorice root, Parsley leaves and root.

Take 3 capsules 3 times daily with a large glass of water.

Available in 100 capsules.

Internal use. Preservative-free.

Capsule.

ARTHRITIS
Homeopathic Complex

A. Nelson & Company Ltd.

Each tablet contains: Berberis vulgaris 6c, Calcarea fluor 6c, Causticum 6c, Dulcamara 6c, Rhus tox 6c, Bryonia 6c, Rhododendron 6c, Nux vomica 6c, Actaea rac 6c, Pulsatilla 6c.

Suck or chew 2 tablets every 2 hours for 6 doses (12 tablets), then 2 tablets 3 times daily until symptoms subside.

72 tablets in blister packs.

Internal use.

Tablet.

Artichoke Juice

W. Schoenenberger

Contains: Pure natural pressed herb and plant juice from organically grown Artichoke plants.

Shake bottle before use. Take 3 or 4 times daily before meals 1 tbsp. diluted in water, milk or tea, one part juice to six parts liquid. For children 1 tsp. full instead of tbsp. Unopened bottle will keep indefinitely: opened, for 6 days.

Amber bottle of 5.5 fl. oz.

Internal use. Organically grown in nearly ideal conditions in the Black Forest & Swabian uplands, where the air is pure. The plants are gathered at the moment when their production of valuable ingredients is at its peak. The juices are extracted by specially designed hydraulic presses that ensure maximum recovery of all essential elements, making certain that not more than 2-3 hours elapse between harvesting, pressing and bottling.

Cellular plant juice.

Artichoke Power™

Nature's Herbs®

Each 475 mg capsule contains: 100 mg. Certified potency® Artichoke extract concentrated and standardized for a minimum of preferred 15 mg. caffeoylquinic acids, synergistically combined in a base of Artichoke powder.

Take 2-3 capsules daily with a large glass of water.

Available in 60 capsules.

Internal use. Preservative-free.

Capsule.

Aspen
Bach Flower Remedy

Bach Flower Remedies® Ltd.

Contains: Populus tremula 5x in 27% grape alcohol solution.

Take 2 drops under the tongue 4 times daily or 2 drops in a small glass of spring water and sip at intervals.

10 ml with dropper.

Internal use.

Liquid.

Astragalus Herbal™

McZand® Herbal Inc.

Contains: Chinese Astragalus (Astragalus membranaceus root) in a base of Codonopsis root, Licorice root, Schisandra berry, Ligustrum root, Ligusticum root, Bai-Shao and Reishi mushroom. Herbs extracted in distilled water, grain alcohol (ethyl alcohol USP) and vegetable glycerine.

Take 2 tablets or 20-40 drops between meals

Available in 59 ml liquid, and 50 and 100 tablets.

Internal use.

Capsule.

Tincture.

Do not take during acute illness.

Astragalus Root

Nature's Herbs®

Each 404 mg capsule contains: Wild countryside® Astragalus root.

Take 2 capsules 3 times daily with a large glass of water preferably at mealtimes.

Available in 100 capsules.

Internal use. Preservative-free

Capsule.

Athletic Tone Capsules
Traditional Yin-Yang Herbals

Flora Manufacturing & Distributing Ltd.

Each 450 mg vegetarian capsule contains: Powdered aqueous extracts of: He shou wu (Polygoni multiflori, radix), Shu di huang (Rehmanniae glutinosae conquitae, radix), Huang qi (Astragali membranacei, radix), Dang shen (Codonopsitis pilosulae, radix), Gou qi zi (Lycii, fructus), Du zhong (Eucommiae ulmoidis, cortex), Mai men dong (Ophiopogonis japonici, tuber), Tu si zi (Cuscutae chinensis, semen),Tian men dong (Asparagi cochinchinensis, tuber), Hong ren sheng (Panax ginseng, radix), Xi yang shen (Panacis quinquefolii, radix), Ling zhi (Ganoderma lucidum), Tian qi (Notoginseng, radix), Wu wei zi (Schisandrae chinensis, semen), Gan cao (Glycyrrhizae uralensis, radix) and purified water.

Take 3-5 capsules daily with liquid for 14 days. Stop for 2 days. Repeat cycle. For maximum results, take 1 hour prior to working out.

90 capsules.

Internal use. No preservatives added. To prevent contamination, do not drink directly from the bottle. After opening, keep refrigerated at all times. Shelf life after opening is 14 days.

Vegicaps®.

Do not use when suffering from a cold, the flu or when digestion is disrupted. Pregnant women should exercise caution when taking this

formula and not exceed the recommended amount.

Athletic Tone Tonic
Traditional Yin-Yang Herbals

Flora Manufacturing and Distributing Ltd.

Each 500 ml contains: He shou wu (Polygoni multiflori, radix), Shu di huang (Rehmanniae glutinosae conquitae, radix, Huang qi (Astragali membranacei, radix), Dang shen (Codonopsitis pilosulae, radix), Gou qi zi (Lycii, fructus), Du zhong (Eucommiae ulmoidis, cortex), Mai men dong (Ophiopogonis japonici, tuber), Tu si zi (Cuscutae chinensis, semen), Tian men dong (Asparagi cochinchinensis, tuber), Hong ren sheng (Panax ginseng, radix), Xi yang shen (Panacis quinquegolii, radix), Ling zhi (Ganoderma lucidum), Tian qi (Notoginseng, radix), Wu wei zi (Schisandrae chinensis, fructus), Gan cao (Glycyrrhizae uralensis, radix).

Take 2 tbsp. 2-3 times daily. Dilute with warm water, if desired. For maximum results, take 1 hour prior to working out. Take formula for 14 days. Stop for 2 days. Repeat cycle.

500 ml.

Internal use. No preservatives added. To prevent contamination, do not drink directly from the bottle. After opening, keep refrigerated at all times. Shelf life after opening is 14 days.

Tonic.

Auxima Calcium
Liquid Supplement

Novartis Nutrition Inc.

Each capful (15 ml) provides 87 mg of elemental Calcium available as Calcium gluconate. Contains: Calciumfed plasmolyzed yeast, Dextrose, Fruit concentrates (Apple, Orange, Grape), Saccharose, Honey, Milk protein, Aromatic plant oil.

Take 1 capful twice daily before morning and evening meals.

Available in 250 ml.

Internal use. Especially suitable for children and the elderly - may be diluted in water.

Liquid.

Visual.

Auxima Fera
Liquid Iron Supplement

Novartis Nutrition Inc.

Each capful (15 ml) provides 16.7 mg of elemental Iron available as ferrous gluconate. Contains: Fruit concentrates (Red grapes, Apples), Ironfed plasmolyzed yeast, Water, Honey, Aromatic plant oils (Orange, Lemon, Anise, Juniper).

Take 1/2 measuring capful twice daily before morning and evening meals.

Available in 250 ml.

- Internal use. Guaranteed not to constipate. May be diluted in water.

- Liquid.

- Visual.

Auxima Magnesium
Liquid Supplement

- **Novartis Nutrition Inc.**

- Each capful (15 ml) provides 114 mg of elemental Magnesium available as Magnesium gluconate. Contains: Magnesiumfed yeast extracts, fruit concentrates (Grapes, Apple), Honey, Lactose, Aromatic oils (Orange, Lemon).

- Take 1 measuring capful (15 ml) twice daily before morning and evening meals.

- Available in 250 ml.

- Internal use. Especially suitable for children and the elderly - may be diluted in water.

- Liquid.

- Visual.

Bakanasan Circu-Caps™
Butcher's Broom Extract

- **Börner GmbH**

- Each capsule contains: 151 mg Gelatin, 75 mg natural Rusci aculeati (Butcher's broom) extract, 2 mg Rosemary oil.

- Take 1 capsule daily.

- Available in 96 capsules.

- Internal use. No preservatives, artificial coloring or flavoring.

- Capsule.

- Visual.

Barley Grass

- **Nature's Herbs®**

- Each 475 mg capsule contains: Premium Barley grass.

- Take 2-3 capsules 3 times daily with a large glass of water.

- Available in 100 capsules.

- Internal use. Preservative-free.

- Capsule.

Basil
Essential Oil

- **Bach-Karooch Ltd.**

- Contains: Ocimum basilicum 100%.

- Two parts Essential oil must be diluted in 98 parts vegetable oil before applying to the skin. Consult Aromatherapy literature for specific methods of use and directions for each oil.

- 10 ml in amber bottle with child-resistant cap and one-drop insert.

- Oil.

- Possible skin irritant.

- Caution: due to high concentration, all oils may be harmful if improperly used! External use only. Avoid during pregnancy.

Bayberry Bark

- **Nature's Herbs®**

- Each capsule contains: Wild countryside® Bayberry bark 450 mg.

- Take 2-3 capsules 3 times daily with a large glass of water.

- Available in 100 capsules.

- Internal use. Preservative-free.

- Capsule.

BE TRANQUIL®
Homeopathic Complex

- **A. Nelson & Company Ltd.**

- Each tablet contains: Kali phos 6c, Arnica montana 6c.

- Dissolve in mouth or chew 2 tablets 3 times daily or when required.

- 72 tablets in blister packs.

- Internal use.

- Tablet.

- If symptoms persist consult a physician.

Bee Health Propolis Capsules

🏠 **Bee Health Propolis**

⚗️ Contains: Propolis, pollen. Propolis contains plant and tree resin, essential oils, waxes and bioflavones.

✋ Take 1-4 capsules daily.

📦 Available in 30 and 90 capsules.

ℹ️ Internal use.

💊 Gelatin capsule.

Bee Health Propolis Lozenges

🏠 **Bee Health Propolis**

⚗️ Contains: Raw Barbados cane sugar, Purified propolis, Raw english honey and Aniseed oil. Propolis contains plant and tree resin, essential oils, waxes and bioflavones.

✋ Use as required.

📦 Available in 4 oz.

ℹ️ Internal use.

Bee Health Propolis Tincture

🏠 **Bee Health Propolis**

⚗️ Contains: Propolis (2:1), Propylene. Propolis contains plant and tree resin, essential oils, waxes and bioflavones.

✋ External: Apply to skin where necessary using a cotton bud moistened with the liquid. Internal: Can be used to drink or gargle, 4-5 drops in half a glass of warm water.

📦 Available in 14 ml and 30 ml.

ℹ️ Internal or external use.

✏️ Tincture.

Bee Pollen

🏠 **Nature's Herbs®**

⚗️ Each 586 mg capsule contains: Wild countryside® Bee pollen.

✋ Take 3 capsules 3 times daily before meals.

📦 Available in 100 capsules.

ℹ️ Internal use. Preservative-free.

💊 Capsule.

Beech

Bach Flower Remedy

🏠 **Bach Flower Remedies® Ltd.**

⚗️ Contains: Fagus sylvatica 5x in 27% grape alcohol solution.

✋ Take 2 drops under the tongue 4 times daily or 2 drops in a small glass of spring water and sip at intervals.

📦 10 ml with dropper.

ℹ️ Internal use.

💧 Liquid.

Belladonna

Homeopathic Remedy

🏠 **A. Nelson & Company Ltd.**

⚗️ Each pillule contains: Belladonna 6c.

✋ Take 2 pillules every 2 hours for the first 6 doses, then 4 times daily for up to 5 days. Pillules should be sucked or chewed and taken between meals.

📦 84 pillules/globules per bottle.

ℹ️ Internal use.

⊘ Pillule/globule.

Benefin Shark Cartilage

🏠 **Lane Labs USA Inc.**

⚗️ Contains: 100% pure Shark cartilage.

✋ Take 1 scoop stirred into water or juice daily or as directed by a health professional.

📦 454 g

ℹ️ Internal use. No added flavors or additives.

🥄 Powder.

Bentonite

🏠 **Inno-Vite Inc.**

⚗️ Contains: Purified water and Bentonite.

Take 1 tbsp. daily in water upon rising.

Available in 500 ml and 1 liter.

Internal use.

Liquid.

Benzoin
Essential Oil

Bach-Karooch Ltd.

Contains: Styrax benzoin 100%.

Two parts Essential oil must be diluted in 98 parts vegetable oil before applying to the skin. Consult Aromatherapy literature for specific methods of use and directions for each oil.

10 ml in amber bottle with child-resistant cap and one-drop insert.

Oil.

Caution: due to high concentration, all oils may be harmful if improperly used! External use only.

Bergamot
Essential Oil

Bach-Karooch Ltd.

Contains: Citrus bergamia 100%.

Two parts Essential oil must be diluted in 98 parts vegetable oil before applying to the skin. Consult Aromatherapy literature for specific methods of use and directions for each oil.

10 ml in amber bottle with child-resistant cap and one-drop insert.

Oil.

Photo sensitization when used on skin.

Caution: due to high concentration, all oils may be harmful if improperly used! External use only.

Betaine Hydrochloride
Digestive Aid

Natural Factors® Nutritional Products Ltd.

Each capsule contains: Betaine hydrochloride 500 mg. Non-medicinal ingredient: Fenugreek seed 100 mg.

Take 2 capsules at mealtime 3 times daily. Maximum daily dose, 6 capsules daily.

Available in 90 and 180 capsules.

Internal use. Contains no artificial preservatives, color, dairy, sweeteners, starch, wheat or yeast.

Capsule.

Visual.

Better Chlorella

Nature's Herbs®

Each 414 mg capsule contains: Better chlorella.

Take 2-3 capsules 3 times daily, preferably at mealtimes.

Available in 100 capsules.

Internal use.

Capsule.

Big Friends Children's Chewable Multi Vitamin

Natural Factors® Nutritional Products Ltd.

Each tablet contains: Beta carotene (Provitamin A) 5000 IU, Vitamin D3 400 IU, Vitamin B-1 (Thiamine hydrochloride) 5 mg, Vitamin B-2 (Riboflavin) 5 mg, Niacinamide 10 mg, Vitamin B-6 (Pyridoxine hydrochloride) 5 mg, Vitamin B-12 (Cyanocobalamin) 10 mcg, d-Pantothenic acid (Calcium pantothenate) 10 mg, Folic acid 0.2 mg, Biotin 10 mcg, Vitamin C 100 mg, Vitamin E (d-alpha Tocopheryl succinate) 25 mg. Lipotropic factors: Choline bitartrate 5 mg, Inositol 5 mg, Minerals: Calcium (citrate) 65 mg, Magnesium (HVP* chelate) 25 mg, Iron (HVP* chelate) 5 mg, Potassium (citrate) 5 mg, Zinc (citrate) 5 mg, Manganese (HVP* chelate) 1 mg. Non-medicinal: Para Amino Benzoic acid 5 mg, Citrus bioflavonoids 5 mg, *Hydrolyzed vegetable protein (rice).

Take 1-2 tablets daily or as directed by a physician.

Available in 60 and 90 tablets.

Internal use. Delicious natural flavors: original jungle juice and mixed fruit flavors.

Chewable tablets.

There is enough iron in this product to seriously harm a child.

📷 Visual.

Big Sky™ Tea Tree Conditioner

🏠 **Prairie Naturals®**

🍵 Contains: Purified Water, Disodium Oleamido Sulfosuccinates, Cocamide DEA/Cocoamido Propyl Purified Water, Cetcaryl Alcohol, Hydrolyzed Grain Protein, Stearalkonium Chloride, Aloe Vera Gel, Ascorbic Acid, Purified Aqueous Extracts of Comfrey, Gravel Root, Lobelia, Spring Horsetail and Lemon Grass, Glycerine, Lecithin, Blended Combinations of Pure Natural Aromatic Oils: Tea Tree, Eucalyptus, Lavender and Clary Sage, Vitamin E Oil, Retinyl Palmitate, D-Panthenol (Pro-Vitamin B5), Jojoba, Grapefruit Seed Extract, Methyl Paraben, Fragrance of Natural Aromatic Oils.

✋ Apply to wet hair. Massage gently into the scalp. Let stand for several minutes, then rinse with lukewarm water.

📖 Available in 125 and 500 ml bottles.

🔲 External use only. Enviro-wise and biodegradable. Not tested on animals.

💧 Conditioner.

Big Sky™ Tea Tree Medicinal Shampoo

🏠 **Prairie Naturals®**

🍵 Contains: Purified water, Disodium oleamido sulfosucinates, Cocoamide DEA/Cocamidopropyl, Purified Water, Cetcaryl Alcohol, Hydrolyzed Grain Protein, Stearalkonium Chloride, Aloe Vera Gel, Ascorbic Acid, Purified Aqueous Extracts of Comfrey, Gravel Root, Lobelia, Spring Horsetail and Lemon Grass, Glycerine, Lecithin, Blended Combinations of Pure Natural Aromatic Oils: Tea Tree, Eucalyptus, Lavender and Clary Sage, Vitamin E Oil, Retinyl Palmitate, D-Panthenol (Pro-Vitamin B5), Jojoba, Grapefruit Seed Extract, Methyl Paraben, Fragrance of Natural Aromatic Oils.

✋ Apply to wet hair. Massage gently into the hair and scalp and let penetrate for several minutes. Rinse with lukewarm water. Follow with a suitable Prairie Naturals Conditioner.

📖 Available in 125 and 500 ml bottles.

🔲 External use only. Enviro-wise and biodegradable. Not tested on animals.

💧 Shampoo.

Bilberry Power®

🏠 **Nature's Herbs®**

🍵 Each capsule contains: 40 mg certified potency Bilberry fruit extract concentrated and standardized for a minimum of preferred 25% anthocyanosides (a unique class of bioflavonoids 10 mg per capsule), synergistically combined in a base of Citrus bioflavonoids, Rutin, and Quercetin.

✋ Take 2 capsules 2 times daily, preferably with meal.

📖 Available in 60 capsules.

🔲 Internal use. Preservative-free.

💊 Capsule.

Bio-Berry OPC-85™ Grape Seed Extract
Plus

🏠 **Flora Manufacturing & Distributing Ltd.**

🍵 Each capsule contains: aqueous/alcohol extracts of: Grape seeds OPC-85™ (98% proanthocyanidins) 50 mg, Bilberries (25% anthocyanins) 1:100 10 mg, in a base of: Cranberry powder (freeze-dried) 290 mg, in Vegicaps® (non-animal source, easily digested capsules). Bio-Berry® contains the authentic Masquelier OPC-85™ Grape seed extract. 350 mg of active ingredients.

✋ Take 1 or 2 capsules twice daily with meals. For maximum absorption, take with berries, fruits or fruit juice.

📖 Available in amber bottles of 60 and 90 capsules.

🔲 Internal use.

💊 Vegetarian capsule.

Bio-K Plus™

Acidophilus Fermented Milk

🏠 **Bio-K+™ International Inc.**

🌿 Water, Milk solids, Modified milk ingredients, Active bacterial cultures. Bio-K has a minimum of 50 billion active acidophilus per 100 g.

📦 100 g

📷 Visual.

Bio-Pectin: Modified Citrus Pectin

🏠 **New Nordic**

🌿 Each tablet contains: Modified citrus pectin (Pexitrus 107™) 500 mg.

🥄 Take 2-4 tablets daily. This dosage is based on an average water consumption of 2 litres daily.

📦 Available in amber bottle 60 and 120 tablets.

Ⅱ Internal use. Modified citrus pectin is a natural complex carbohydrate extracted from a selection of five citrus fruit pulps. Contains soluble fiber. Bio-Pectin (Pexitrus™) tablets contain the original modified citrus pectin known as Pexitrus 107.™ Pexitrus 107 was developed in Copenhagen. The pectin is a purified carbohydrate obtained by aqueous extraction of edible material from the peel of lemon, lime, orange and grapefruit. It consists mainly of galacturonic acid and galacturonic acid methyl ester units forming linear polysaccharide chains. The parts of the fruit used are flavedo, albedo, lamella and the core. The modification procedures are very important to the final characteristics and quality of the modified citrus pectin.

Bio-Strath Herbal Yeast Food Supplements

🏠 **Bio-Strath AG®**

🌿 100% plasmolysed herbal yeast (filtrate).

 Take 30 drops with a small amount of water, 3 times daily before meals.
Children: 1/2 of adult dosage.

📦 Also available in drops.

Ⅱ No synthetically produced additives. Non-habit forming; can be taken continuously. Storage life: 5 years, naturally preserved.

💧 Liquid.

⊘ Tablet.

🍼 Tonic.

📷 Visual.

Black Cohosh Root

🏠 **Nature's Herbs®**

🌿 Each 545 mg capsule contains: Wild countryside® Black cohosh root.

🥄 Take 1 capsule 3 times daily with a large glass of water.

📦 Available in 100 capsules.

Ⅱ Internal use. Preservative-free.

▭ Capsule.

Black Radish Juice

🏠 **W. Schoenenberger**

🌿 Contains: Pure natural pressed herb and plant juice from organically grown Black radish plants.

🥄 Shake bottle before use. Take 3 or 4 times daily before meals 1 tbsp. diluted in water, milk or tea, one part juice to six parts liquid. For children 1 tsp. instead of tbsp. Unopened bottle will keep indefinitely: opened, for 6 days.

📦 Amber bottle of 5.5 fl. oz.

Ⅱ Internal use. Organically grown in nearly ideal conditions in the Black Forest & Swabian uplands, where the air is pure. The plants are gathered at the moment when their production of valuable ingredients is at its peak. The juices are extracted by specially designed hydraulic presses that ensure maximum recovery of all essential elements, making certain that not more than 2-3 hours elapse between harvesting, pressing and bottling.

💧 Cellular plant juice.

Black Seed-500

🏠 **Kare & Hope Inc.**

🌿 Each capsule contains: Black seed 500 mg.

Take 2 capsules twice daily or as recommended by a health care professional.

100 capsules.

No added sugar, salt, preservatives or any artificial chemicals.

Capsule.

Black Walnut Hulls

Nature's Herbs®

Each 495 mg capsule contains: Wild countryside® Black walnut hulls.

Take 2 capsules 3 times daily with a large glass of water.

Available in 100 capsules.

Internal use. Preservative-free.

Capsule.

Blessed Thistle

Nature's Herbs®

Each capsule contains: Certified organically grown Blessed thistle herb 360 mg.

Take 2 capsules 3 times daily with a large glass of water.

Available in 100 capsules.

Internal use. Preservative-free.

Capsule.

Blessed Thistle Combination

Nature's Herbs®

Each capsule contains: Blessed thistle, Red raspberry leaves, Goldenseal root, Ginger root, Cramp bark, Uva ursi leaves, Marshmallow root, Cayenne, Squawvine, and False unicorn root.

Take 2-3 capsules 3 times daily with a large glass of water.

Available in 100 capsules.

Internal use. Preservative-free.

Capsule.

Boldocynara® N

A. Vogel

Bioforce AG

Contains: Fresh organically grown Artichoke herb, Milk thistle fruit, fresh wild Dandelion root and herb, Boldo leaf, fresh organically grown Peppermint herb and non-medicinal

Take 10-15 drops 3 times daily take in a small amount of water after meals. Salivate before swallowing.

Available in 50 ml.

Internal use.

Tincture.

 May have a slight laxative effect which can be resolved by a reduction in dosage.

Contraindicated during nursing and high risk pregnancy.

Born Again® Glucosamine Super Pain Relieving Cream
with Capsaicin

Alvin Last, Inc.

Contains: Capsicum oleoresin (Capsaicin 0.025%), Aloe vera gel, N-Acetyl-D-Glucosamine, Soybean oil, Stearic acid, Cetyl alcohol, Triethanolamine, Glycerin, Arnica montana extract, Willow bark extract (white), Tocopherol (Vitamin E), Ascorbic acid (Vitamin C), Methylparaben, Propylparaben. Every 1/2 tsp. provides 250 mg of Glucosamine.

Adults and children 2 years of age and older: apply to affected area not more than 3 to 4 times daily.

Available in 2 oz.

External use only. Fragrance free. Not tested on animals. For children under 2 years of age, consult a doctor or orthopedic physician.

Cream.

Avoid contact with the eyes and mucous membranes. If condition worsens, or if symptoms persist for more than 7 days or clear up and occur again within a few days, consult your doctor. Do not apply to wounds or damaged skin. Do not bandage tightly.

Born Again® Glucosamine Super Pain Relieving Roll-On
with Capsaicin

Alvin Last, Inc.

Contains: Capsicum oleoresin (Capsaicin 0.025%), Aloe vera gel, N-Acetyl-D-Glucosamine, Soybean oil, Glycerin, Arnica montana extract, Willow bark extract (white), Stearic acid, Triethanolamine, Cetyl alcohol, Tocopherol (Vitamin E), Ascorbic acid (Vitamin C), Methylparaben, Propylparaben. Every 1/2 tsp. provides 250 mg of Glucosamine.

Adults and children 2 years of age and older apply to affected area not more than 3–4 times daily.
For children under 2 years of age, consult a doctor or orthopedic physician.

Available in 1.5 fl. oz.

External use. Not tested on animals. Fragrance free. Every 1/2 tsp. provides 250 mg of Glucosamine.

Roll-on.

Avoid contact with the eyes and mucous membranes. If condition worsens, or if symptoms persist for more than 7 days or clear up and occur again within a few days, consult a doctor. Do not apply to wounds or damaged skin. Do not bandage tightly.

Born Again® Vaginal Moisturizing Gel

with Wild Yam Extract and Vitamin E

Alvin Last, Inc.

Contains: Water, Wild yam extract, Glycerin, Sodium alginate, Tocopheryl acetate, Methylparaben, Citric acid (added for pH balance).

Squeeze out a small amount of gel to cover fingertip and apply to the vaginal opening and external area as needed.

Available in 1.5 oz.

External use. Greaseless. Fragrance free. Water-based. Non-staining. Not tested on animals. Does not contain animal by-products.

Gel.

This product is not a contraceptive. Avoid contact with eyes.

Born Again® Wild Yam Cream

with Vitamin E

Alvin Last, Inc.

Contains: Wild yam extract, Aloe vera gel, Soybean oil, Stearic acid, Cetyl alcohol, Triethanolamine, Tocopheryl acetate, Glycerin, Methylparaben, Propylparaben.

Twice a day rub 1/4 to 1/2 tsp. of cream into the soft parts of the body: belly, breasts, or under the upper arms.

Available in 2 oz.

External use. Fragrance free. Not tested on animals.

Cream.

Born Again® Wild Yam Meno-Herbs™

with Mexican Wild Yam and other Botanicals

Alvin Last, Inc.

Each 725 mg tablet contains: Wild yam (root part) 280 mg, Black cohosh (root part) 252 mg, Squaw vine (leaf part) 168 mg, Raspberry leaf 168 mg, Licorice (root part) 168 mg, Siberian ginseng (root part) 168 mg, Dong quai (root part) 112 mg, Chaste tree (Berry pan) 56 mg, False unicorn (root part) 28 mg. Additional ingredients: Stearic acid, Magnesium stearate, Guar gum and Silica as excipients.

Take 2 tablets daily. In acute situations, increase dosage to 2 tablets three times daily. Stop after one week. Rest one day. Repeat if needed.

Available in 90 tablets.

Internal use.

Tablet.

Bromelain

Albi Imports Ltd.

Each capsule contains: Bromelain 500 mg. Each gram of this extra strength Bromelain extract contains 1000 GDU (Gelatin digesting units) and 1500 MCU (Milk clotting units) of enzyme activity.

Take 1 or more capsules, as desired, at mealtime with water or juice.

Available in 100 and 200 capsules.

Internal use.

- Capsule.

- May be irritating to people affected by irritable bowel syndrome.

Bromelain 500 mg
Extra Strength

- Natural Factors® Nutritional Products Ltd.

- Each capsule contains: Bromelain 500 mg. With vegetable grade Magnesium stearate (used as a lubricant). Note: Each gram of this extra strength Bromelain extract contains 1000 GDU and 1500 MCU of enzyme activity. *GDU - Gelatin Digesting Units. MCU - Milk Clotting Units.

- Take 1 or more capsules at mealtime.

- Available in 90 and 180 capsules.

- Internal use. Contains no artificial preservatives, color, dairy, sweeteners, starch, wheat or yeast.

- Capsule.

- Visual.

Bronc-Ease®

- Nature's Herbs®

- Each capsule contains: Slippery elm bark 150 mg, White pine 75 mg, Horehound 75 mg, Mullein leaves 37.5 mg, Marshmallow root 37.5 mg, Lobelia 37.5 mg.

- Adults and children over 12 years: take 2-3 capsules 3 times daily; children 5-11 years take 1-2 capsules daily. Under 4 years; as directed by physician.

- Available in 100 capsules.

- Internal use. Preservative-free.

- Capsule.

- Do not take for persistent or chronic cough. Do not give to children under 2 years of age. Consult a doctor if you have high blood pressure, heart disease, diabetes, or are pregnant or nursing.

Bryonia
Homeopathic Remedy

- A. Nelson & Company Ltd.

- Each pillule contains: Bryonia alba 6c.

- Take 2 pillules every 2 hours for the first 6 doses, then 4 times daily for up to 5 days. Pillules should be sucked or chewed and taken between meals.

- 84 pillules/globules per bottle.

- Internal use.

- Pillule/globule.

Burdock Root

- Nature's Herbs®

- Each 475 mg capsule contains: Certified organically grown Burdock root.

- Take 3 capsules 3 times daily with a large glass of water.

- Available in 100 capsules.

- Internal use. Preservative-free.

- Capsule.

Butcher's Broom Root

- Nature's Herbs®

- Each 475 mg capsule contains: Wild Countryside® Butcher's broom root.

- Take 2-3 capsules 3 times daily with a large glass of water.

- Available in 100 capsules.

- Internal use. Preservative-free.

- Capsule.

C Extra 500 mg
Plus 500 mg Bioflavonoids

- Natural Factors® Nutritional Products Ltd.

- Each tablet contains: Vitamin C 500 mg. Non-medicinal ingredients: Bioflavonoid complex (lemon, orange, grapefruit) 500 mg, Rutin 50 mg, Rosehips 50 mg, Hesperidin 25 mg.

- Take 1-3 tablets daily or as directed by a physician.

- Available in 60, 90, 180 and 360 tablets.

- Internal use. Contains no artificial preservatives, color, dairy, sweeteners, starch, wheat or yeast.

⊘ Tablet.

📷 Visual.

C Extra 500 mg
Plus 250 mg Bioflavonoids

🏠 **Natural Factors®
Nutritional Products Ltd.**

⚗ Each capsule contains:
Vitamin C 500 mg. Non-medicinal ingredients: Bioflavonoid complex (lemon, orange, grapefruit) 250 mg, Rutin 50 mg, Rosehips 25 mg, Hesperidin 25 mg.

✍ Take 1-3 capsules daily or as directed by a physician.

📖 Available in 60, 90 and 180 capsules.

🔳 Internal use. Contains no artificial preservatives, color, dairy, sweeteners, starch, wheat or yeast.

▭ Capsule.

📷 Visual.

C.L.A.™ (U.S.)
Conjugated Linoleic Acid

🏠 **EAS**

⚗ Each capsule contains: 1000 mg vegetable oil with 60% conjugated Linoleic acid (GLA) and 40% other monounsaturated and saturated fatty acids. 0.02% TBHQ (antioxidant) has been added to preserve freshness.

✍ Take 2 capsules 3 times daily with meals.

📖 Available in 90 softgel capsules.

🔳 Internal use. A mixture of positional and geometric isomers of linoleic acid with conjugated double bonds.

▭ Softgel capsule.

📷 Visual.

C Serum™

🏠 **Nutraceutics Corporation**

⚗ Contains: L Ascorbic acid, Maxogenol™ (dermal active antioxidant complex).

✍ Use twice daily. Apply after cleansing.

📖 Available in 1 oz. / 30 ml cream.

🔳 External use only.

Cajeput
Essential Oil

🏠 **Bach-Karooch Ltd.**

⚗ Contains: Melaleuca cajeputi 100%.

✍ Two parts Essential oil must be diluted in 98 parts vegetable oil before applying to the skin. Consult Aromatherapy literature for specific methods of use and directions for each oil.

📖 10 ml in amber bottle with child-resistant cap and one-drop insert.

💧 Oil.

⚠ Caution: due to high concentration, all oils may be harmful if improperly used!
External use only.

Cal'dophilus Super Strength
FOS

🏠 **Natural Factors®
Nutritional Products Ltd.**

⚗ Each capsule contains: 6 billion active cells of the following specially cultured strains of probiotics: L. rhamnosus 50% 3.00 billion, L. casei 30% 1.80 billion, L. acidophilus 10% 0.60 billion, B. longum 10% 0.60 billion to maintain healthful balance. FOS (Fructooligosaccharides: naturally occurring complex fructose molecules derived from chicory root) 200 mg. These micro-organisms are in a base of powdered Malto-dextrin, Calcium gluconate, Pectin, Magnesium stearate (used as a lubricant), Ascorbic acid in a gelatin capsule.

✍ Take 3 capsules daily at mealtime.

📖 Available in 60, 90 and 180 capsules.

🔳 Internal use. Contains no artificial preservatives, color, corn, dairy, soya, starch or yeast. Non-dairy.

▭ Capsule.

📷 Visual.

Calaguala Fern and Cade Tar
Scalp Treatment Shampoo

🏠 **Aubrey Organics®**

⚗ Contains: Coconut and corn oil soap, organic Aloe vera gel, Quillaya bark extract 10%, Calaguala fern extract (Polypodium leucotomos) 5%, Yucca root extract 5%, Evening primrose oil 2%, White pine bark extract 2%,

Cade tar 1%, Citrus seed extract with Vitamins A, C and E, and oil of lemon peel.

Dampen hair. Apply shampoo, work into lather, rinse. Repeat and rinse well.

Available in 8 oz.

External use. No coal tar.

Shampoo.

Calc. Carb.

Homeopathic Remedy

A. Nelson & Company Ltd.

Each pillule contains: Calcarea carbonica 6c.

Take 2 pillules every 2 hours for the first 6 doses, then 4 times daily for up to 5 days. Pillules should be sucked or chewed and taken between meals.

84 pillules/globules per bottle.

Internal use.

Pillule/globule.

Calc. Fluor.

Homeopathic Remedy

A. Nelson & Company Ltd.

Each pillule contains: Calcarea fluorica 6c.

Take 2 pillules every 2 hours for the first 6 doses, then 4 times daily for up to 5 days. Pillules should be sucked or chewed and taken between meals.

84 pillules/globules per bottle.

Internal use.

Pillule/globule.

Calc. Phos.

Homeopathic Remedy

A. Nelson & Company Ltd.

Each pillule contains: Calcarea phosphorica 6c.

Take 2 pillules every 2 hours for the first 6 doses, then 4 times daily for up to 5 days. Pillules should be sucked or chewed and taken between meals.

84 pillules/globules per bottle.

Internal use.

Pillule/globule.

Calcium 350 mg

Citrate

Natural Factors® Nutritional Products Ltd.

Each tablet contains: elemental Calcium (citrate) 350 mg.

Take 1-4 tablets daily or as directed by a physician.

Available in 60 and 90 tablets.

Internal use. Contains no artificial preservatives, color, dairy, sweeteners, starch, wheat or yeast.

Tablet.

Visual.

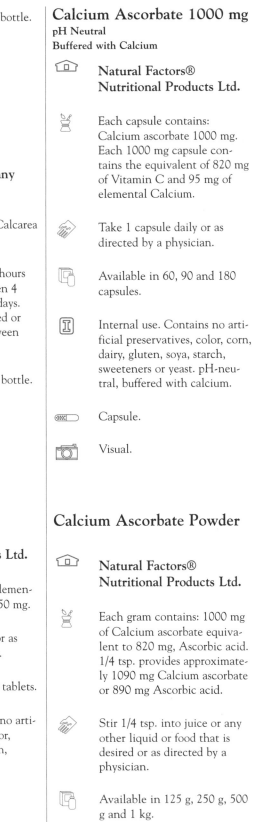

Calcium Ascorbate 1000 mg

pH Neutral
Buffered with Calcium

Natural Factors® Nutritional Products Ltd.

Each capsule contains: Calcium ascorbate 1000 mg. Each 1000 mg capsule contains the equivalent of 820 mg of Vitamin C and 95 mg of elemental Calcium.

Take 1 capsule daily or as directed by a physician.

Available in 60, 90 and 180 capsules.

Internal use. Contains no artificial preservatives, color, corn, dairy, gluten, soya, starch, sweeteners or yeast. pH-neutral, buffered with calcium.

Capsule.

Visual.

Calcium Ascorbate Powder

Natural Factors® Nutritional Products Ltd.

Each gram contains: 1000 mg of Calcium ascorbate equivalent to 820 mg, Ascorbic acid. 1/4 tsp. provides approximately 1090 mg Calcium ascorbate or 890 mg Ascorbic acid.

Stir 1/4 tsp. into juice or any other liquid or food that is desired or as directed by a physician.

Available in 125 g, 250 g, 500 g and 1 kg.

Internal use. Contains no artificial preservatives, color, dairy, sweeteners, starch, wheat or yeast.

Powder.

Visual.

Calcium & Magnesium
Citrate Plus

Natural Factors®
Nutritional Products Ltd.

Each capsule contains: Elemental Calcium (citrate/malate) 125 mg, Magnesium (citrate/oxide) 125 mg, Potassium (citrate) 10 mg, Zinc (citrate) 5 mg, Manganese (citrate) 1 mg.

Take 3 capsules daily or as directed by a physician.

Available in 90 and 180 capsules.

Internal use. Contains no artificial preservatives, color, dairy, sweeteners, starch, wheat or yeast.

Capsule.

Visual.

Calcium & Magnesium
Chelated Plus C, Potassium + Zinc

Natural Factors®
Nutritional Products Ltd.

Each tablet contains: elemental Calcium (HVP* chelate/carbonate) 350 mg, Magnesium (HVP* chelate/oxide) 175 mg,

Potassium (citrate) 10 mg, Zinc (citrate) 5 mg, Vitamin C 200 mg. Non-medicinal ingredient: Silica 5 mg.
*Hydrolyzed vegetable protein (sourced from rice).

Take 2 tablets daily or as directed by a physician.

Available in 90 and 180 tablets.

Internal use. Contains no artificial preservatives, color, dairy, sweeteners, starch, wheat or yeast.

Tablet.

Visual.

Calcium & Magnesium
Plus D + Betaine

Natural Factors®
Nutritional Products Ltd.

Each capsule contains: elemental Calcium (carbonate) 250 mg, Magnesium (oxide) 125 mg, Vitamin D3 100 IU, Non-medicinal ingredient: Betaine hydrochloride 60 mg.

Take 1-4 capsules daily or as directed by a physician.

Available in 90 and 180 capsules.

Internal use. Contains no artificial preservatives, color, dairy, sweeteners, starch, wheat or yeast.

Capsule (easy to swallow).

Visual.

Calcium & Magnesium Citrate
Plus Potassium + Zinc

Natural Factors®
Nutritional Products Ltd.

Each tablet contains: elemental Calcium (citrate/carbonate) 250 mg, Magnesium (citrate/oxide) 250 mg, Potassium (citrate) 20 mg, Zinc (citrate) 5 mg. Non-medicinal ingredients: Betaine hydrochloride 50 mg, Silica 5 mg.

Take 2 tablets daily or as directed by a physician.

Available in 60, 90 and 180 tablets.

Internal use. Contains no artificial preservatives, color, dairy, sweeteners, starch, wheat or yeast.

Tablet.

Visual.

Calcium & Magnesium Citrate
Plus D3

Natural Factors®
Nutritional Products Ltd.

Each capsule contains: elemental Calcium (citrate/malate) 125 mg, Magnesium (citrate/oxide) 125 mg, Manganese (citrate) 1 mg, Potassium (citrate) 10 mg, Zinc (citrate) 5 mg, Vitamin D3 100 IU.

Take 3 capsules daily or as directed by a physician.

Available in 90 and 180 capsules.

Internal use. Contains no artificial preservatives, color, dairy, sweeteners, starch, wheat or yeast. Adult use only.

Capsule.

Visual.

Calcium & Magnesium Citrate Plus D

Natural Factors® Nutritional Products Ltd.

Each tablet contains: Elemental Calcium (citrate/carbonate) 250 mg, Elemental Magnesium (citrate/oxide) 250 mg, Elemental Potassium (citrate) 20 mg, Elemental Zinc (citrate) 5 mg, Elemental Manganese (citrate) 1 mg, Vitamin D3 100 IU, Non-medicinal ingredients: Betaine hydrochloride 50 mg, Silica 5 mg.

Take 2 tablets daily or as directed by a physician.

Available in 60, 90 and 180 tablets.

Internal use. Contains no artificial preservatives, color, dairy, sweeteners, starch, wheat or yeast.

Tablet.

Visual.

Calendula Cream
Homeopathic Cream

A. Nelson & Company Ltd.

Contains: Extract of organically grown Calendula officinalis

1x 9% in a base of almond oil, avocado oil and cocoa butter.

Apply to affected areas.

27 g tube.

External use. Organic. Not tested on animals.

Cream.

Avoid contact with eyes. If symptoms persist, consult a physician.

Calendula/Flax Oil "E.F.A." Balm
Flora Herbal Cream

Flora Manufacturing & Distributing Ltd.

Contains: Distilled water, certified organic unrefined Flax oil, Glyceryl-stearate*, Emulsifying wax*, Calendula extract, Glycerine, Glucose moisturizer, Phenonip (cosmetic preservative), Vitamin E, Lavender oil. *Naturally derived from coconut.

Apply daily for smooth and healthy looking skin.

60 ml in opaque jar.

External use only.

Cream.

Calming Herbal™

McZand® Herbal Inc.

Each ml contains: Valerian root 193 mg, Passion flower herb 45.0 mg, Scullcap herb

39.0 mg, Chamomile flowers 39.0 mg. Non-medicinal: Schizandra fruit 19.0 mg, Oatstraw 26.0 mg, Bupleurum root 26.0 mg, Pueria root 13.0 mg. All ingredients are present as 1:2.5 extracts in 30% alcohol.

Take 35-45 drops or 2 capsules between meals 3 times daily.

Available in 59 ml liquid and 60 capsules.

Internal use.

Capsule.

Tincture.

May cause drowsiness.

Camomile Extract

Nature's Herbs®

Contains: EuroQuality® extract of Chamomile, standardized for .5% Essential oil, 6 g, in pure alpine spring water. Pure grain alcohol, 20% by volume.

Take 10-30 drops 3 times daily with water or juice. Shake well before use.

Available in 1 oz (30 ml).

Internal use.

Tincture.

Camomile Tincture

Salus-Haus

Each 10 g tincture contains: 10 g extract derived from 2.0 g Camomile blossoms. Alcohol content: 32% v/v.

Unless otherwise directed, take 5-10 drops diluted in a small amount of liquid 3 times daily.

Available in 50 ml, includes a dropper.

Internal use. Salus herbal tinctures are made in accordance with strictest health food principles, using natural ingredients only.

Tincture.

Camphor White
Essential Oil

Bach-Karooch Ltd.

Contains: Cinnamomum camphora 100%.

Two parts Essential oil must be diluted in 98 parts vegetable oil before applying to the skin. Consult Aromatherapy literature for specific methods of use and directions for each oil.

10 ml in amber bottle with child-resistant cap and one-drop insert.

Oil.

Caution: due to high concentration, all oils may be harmful if improperly used! External use only.

CANDIDA-AWAY®™
Homeopathic Complex

A. Nelson & Company Ltd.

Each tablet contains: Candida albicans 6c, Kreosotum 6c, Thuja occidentalis 6c.

Dissolve in mouth or chew 2 tablets 3 times daily until symptoms subside.

72 tablets in blister packs.

Internal use.

Tablet.

Cantharis
Homeopathic Remedy

A. Nelson & Company Ltd.

Each pillule contains: Cantharis 6c.

Take 2 pillules every 2 hours for the first 6 doses, then 4 times daily for up to 5 days. Pillules should be sucked or chewed and taken between meals.

84 pillules/globules per bottle.

Internal use.

Pillule/globule.

Caprillian Plus

Nutra Research International

Each capsule contains: Capryllic acid 150 mg, Black walnut concentrate 150 mg, 200 million units of Carrot acidophilus, 185 mg combination of Garlic, Chaparral, Dulse, Burdock root.

Take 1-3 capsules on an empty stomach with 1 to 2 glasses of warm water.

Will be more effective with a diet low in dairy, meat, fruits, white flour and sugar.

Capsule.

May cause loose stools if taken with meals. Available in 90 capsules.

Carbo. Veg.
Homeopathic Remedy

A. Nelson & Company Ltd.

Each pillule contains: Carbo vegetabilis 6c.

Take 2 pillules every 2 hours for the first 6 doses, then 4 times daily for up to 5 days. Pillules should be sucked or chewed and taken between meals.

84 pillules/globules per bottle.

Internal use.

Pillule/globule.

Carrot Seed
Essential Oil

Bach-Karooch Ltd.

Contains: Daucus carota 100%.

Two parts Essential oil must be diluted in 98 parts vegetable oil before applying to the skin. Consult Aromatherapy literature for specific methods of use and directions for each oil.

10 ml in amber bottle with child-resistant cap and one-drop insert.

Oil.

Caution: due to high concentration, all oils may be harmful if improperly used! External use only.

Cascara Sagrada

Nature's Herbs®

Each capsule contains: Cascara sagrada bark 450 mg.

Adults and children 12 years of age and over: take 2 capsules at bedtime. Children 2-12 years take 1 capsule at bedtime.

Available in 100 capsules.

Internal use. Preservative-free.

Capsule.

Do not use if you have abdominal pain, nausea, fever or vomiting, rectal bleeding or failure to have a bowel movement after the use of the laxative. If pregnant or nursing use on advice of doctor only. Do not take for more than one week unless advised by a physician. Overuse or extended use may cause dependence for bowel function. Do not take a laxative within two hours of another medicine because the desired effect of the other medicine may be reduced.

Cat's Claw

Inno-Vite Inc.

Each capsule contains: Cat's claw (bark) powder 500 mg.

Take 2 capsules 3 times daily.

Available in 90 capsules.

Internal use.

Capsule.

Cat's Claw

Nature's Herbs®

Each 500 mg capsule contains: Wild countryside® Cat's claw bark.

Take 1-2 capsules 3 times daily.

Available in 50 capsules.

Internal use.

Capsule.

Do not use if you are pregnant or nursing.

Cat's Claw Extract
200 mg

Natural Factors® Nutritional Products Ltd.

Each capsule contains: Cat's claw bark extract (Uncaria tomentosa) 200 mg standardized to contain 3% alkaloids in a base of 200 mg of Cat's claw powder in a gelatin capsule with vegetable grade Magnesium stearate (used as a lubricant).

Take 1 capsule daily or as directed by a physician.

Available in 60 and 90 capsules.

Internal use. Contains no artificial preservatives, color, dairy, sweeteners, starch, wheat or yeast.

Capsule.

Visual.

Cayenne

Albi Imports Ltd.

Each capsule contains: 500 mg cayenne powder.

Take 1–3 capsules daily.

Available in 90, 180 and 500 capsules.

Internal use. Available in three heat unit strengths to best meet individual needs. Cool Capsaicin is 9,000 heat units, mild cayenne is 30,000, and hot cayenne 50,000 heat units.

Capsule.

Not recommended for individuals with peptic ulcers, gastritis or inflammatory bowel conditions.

Visual.

Cayenne

Nature's Herbs®

Each 455 mg capsule contains: Premium Cayenne standardized at 40,000 STU's.

Take 2-3 capsules 3 times daily with a large glass of water.

Available in 100 capsules.

Internal use. Preservative-free.

Capsule.

Cayenne Power Herb®

Nature's Herbs®

Each capsule contains: 450 mg Certified potency Cayenne standardized at 100,000 STU's.

Take 1 capsule 3 times daily, preferably right before meals with a large glass of cold water.

Available in 60 capsules.

Internal use. Preservative-free.

Capsule.

Cedar Berry Combination

Nature's Herbs®

Each 475 mg capsule contains: Cedar berries, Licorice root, Uva ursi leaves, Goldenseal root, Mullein leaves, and Cayenne.

Take 2-3 capsules 3 times daily with a large glass of water.

Available in 100 capsules.

Internal use. Preservative-free.

Capsule.

Cedarwood Virginian
Essential Oil

Bach-Karooch Ltd.

Contains: Juniperus virginiana 100%.

Two parts Essential oil must be diluted in 98 parts vegetable oil before applying to the skin. Consult Aromatherapy literature for specific methods of use and directions for each oil.

10 ml in amber bottle with child-resistant cap and one-drop insert.

Oil.

Possible skin irritant.

Caution: due to high concentration, all oils may be harmful if improperly used!
External use only. Avoid during pregnancy.

Celery Seed

Nature's Herbs®

Each 505 mg capsule contains: Celery seed powder.

Take 3 capsules 3 times daily, preferably before meals.

Available in 100 capsules.

Internal use. Preservative-free.

Capsule.

This product should not be used by people with kidney disorders. Not intended for use during pregnancy. Do not use if you are allergic to celery. People with fair skin should

not overexpose themselves to strong sunlight while taking this product due to the photo-sensitizing nature of this plant.

Cell Respirate

Klaire Laboratories, Inc., USA & Europe

Each capsule contains: L-Carnitine (Fumarate) 80 mg, Malic acid 70 mg, Inosine 60 mg, Alpha-Ketoglutaric acid 50 mg, Dimethylglycine 50 mg, p-Aminobenzoic acid 50 mg, Coenzyme Q10 30 mg, Ascorbic acid (Magnesium ascorbate) 24 mg, Niacinamide 15 mg, D-Calcium pantothenate 10 mg, Magnesium (ascorbate) 3 mg, Manganese (Manganese sulfate) 2 mg, Vitamin B2 (Riboflavin) 2 mg. Vitamin B1 (Thiamine HCl) 2 mg, Selenium (Selenomethionine) 25 mcg. Added ingredients: Potassium phosphate (Monobasic), Potassium phosphate (Dibasic) and L-leucine.

Take 1 or 2 capsules daily or as directed by a physician. Buffering agents used to assure a pH of 5.

Available in 60 capsules.

Internal use.

Capsule.

Cell-Life® Defence

Nu-Life Nutrition Ltd.™

Each caplet contains: Beta-carotene (Provitamin A) 15,000 IU, Vitamin E (d-alpha Tocopherol succinate) 200 IU,

Vitamin C (Calcium ascorbate) 350 mg, Vitamin B2 (Riboflavin, Ribo 5' phosphate) 25 mg, Zinc (citrate, fumerate, malate, glutarate, succinate) 15 mg, Copper (Malate, fumerate, citrate, succinate, glutarate) 0.5 mg, Manganese (Citrate, malate, glutarate, succinate) 2 mg, Chromium (Citrate, malate, fumerate, glutarate, succinate) 25 mcg, Selenium (Citrate, fumerate, glutarate, succinate) 100 mcg. Lipotropic factors: Methionine 25 mg. Non-Medicinal: L-Cysteine 35 mg, Alginic acid 25 mg, Quercetin 30 mg, L-glutathione (99% reduced) 5 mg, Rosemary extract 1:4 20 mg, Bilberry extract 2 mg, Red cabbage extract 2 mg, Red wine concentrate 5mg, Grape seed extract 5 mg, Chinese green tea extract 10 mg. In a non-medicinal base of Garlic, Capsicum and Echinacea.

Take 2 caplets daily, with meals, or as directed by a health professional.

60 cpalets.

Internal use. Full spectrum antioxidant formula. Free of allergens found in the following foods: milk, corn, yeast, citrus and egg. Contains no preservatives, artificial colors, starch or sugar.

Caplet.

Centaury
Bach Flower Remedy

Bach Flower Remedies® Ltd.

Contains: Centarium umbellatum 5x in 27% grape alcohol solution.

Take 2 drops under the tongue 4 times daily or 2 drops in a small glass of spring water and sip at intervals.

10 ml with dropper.

Internal use.

Liquid.

Cerato
Bach Flower Remedy

Bach Flower Remedies® Ltd.

Contains: Ceratostigma willmotiana 5x in 27% grape alcohol solution.

Take 2 drops under the tongue 4 times daily or 2 drops in a small glass of spring water and sip at intervals.

10 ml with dropper.

Internal use.

Liquid.

Chamomile Blue
Essential Oil

Bach-Karooch Ltd.

Contains: Matricaria chamomillia 100%.

Two parts Essential oil must be diluted in 98 parts vegetable oil before applying to the skin. Consult Aromatherapy literature for specific methods of use and directions for each oil.

10 ml in amber bottle with child-resistant cap and one-drop insert.

Oil.

Possible dermatitis in some individuals.

Caution: due to high concentration, all oils may be harmful if improperly used! External use only.

Chamomile Flowers

Nature's Herbs®

Each 354 mg capsule contains: Premium Chamomile flowers.

Take 2-3 capsules 3 times daily with a full glass or water.

Available in 100 capsules.

Internal use.

Capsule.

Chamomile Morocco
Essential Oil

Bach-Karooch Ltd.

Contains: Ormenis multicaulis 100%.

Two parts Essential oil must be diluted in 98 parts vegetable oil before applying to the skin. Consult Aromatherapy literature for specific methods of use and directions for each oil.

10 ml in amber bottle with child-resistant cap and one-drop insert.

Oil.

Caution: due to high concentration, all oils may be harmful if improperly used! External use only.

Chamomile Roman
Essential Oil

🏠 **Bach-Karooch Ltd.**

⚗️ Contains: Anthemis nobilis 100%.

🤲 Two parts Essential oil must be diluted in 98 parts vegetable oil before applying to the skin. Consult Aromatherapy literature for specific methods of use and directions for each oil.

📦 10 ml in amber bottle with child-resistant cap and one-drop insert.

💧 Oil.

⚠️ Caution: due to high concentration, all oils may be harmful if improperly used! External use only.

Changes for Men®

🏠 **McZand® Herbal Inc.**

⚗️ Contains: Saw palmetto (Serenoa repens berry) in a base of Nettle root, Pygeum bark, Horsetail herb, Coptis root, Cuscuta seed, Scutellaria root, Marshmallow root, Hawthorn berry, Licorice root and Bupleurum root. Herbs extracted in distilled water, grain alcohol (ethyl alcohol USP) and vegetable glycerine.

🤲 Take 2 capsules or 20-40 drops between meals 2-3 times daily.

📦 Available in 59 ml liquid and 60 capsules.

🔢 Internal use. A herbal formula to support the changing needs of men over the age of 35.

💊 Capsule.

💧 Tincture.

Changes for Women®

🏠 **McZand® Herbal Inc.**

⚗️ Each capsule contains: Calcium chelate (50 mg), Magnesium chelate (25 mg), Pantothenic acid (25 mg), Vitamin E (25 IU), Dong quai root, Vitex agnus-castus berry, Bai-Shao, Polyporus sclerotum, Bupleurum root, Astragalus root, Atractylodes root, Moutan root bark, Gardenia fruit, Ginger root, Oatstraw herb, Licorice root, Nettle leaf, Selenium chelate (25 mcg), Peppermint leaf, Scullcap herb, Chromium chelate (25 mcg) and Boron chelate (10 mcg). Herbs are prepared as a powdered extract (5:1) to enhance potency.

🤲 Take 2 capsules or 20-40 drops between meals 1-3 times daily.

📦 Available in 59 ml liquid and 60 capsules.

🔢 Internal use. Herbal nutritional supplement to support the changing needs of women over the age of 35.

💊 Capsule.

💧 Tincture.

⚠️ Do not take during pregnancy or during the menstrual cycle.

Chasteberry-Power™

🏠 **Nature's Herbs®**

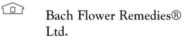

⚗️ Each capsule contains: 100 mg. Certified potency ChasteBerry fruit and seeds (Vitex agnus castus) concentrated and standardized for a minimum of preferred 1.1% glycosides in a synergistic base of Wild countryside® Dong quai root, Siberian ginseng, Gelatin.

🤲 Take 2 capsules with both morning and evening meals.

📦 Available in 60 capsules.

🔢 Internal use.

💊 Capsule.

⚠️ Do not consume Dong quai (Angelica sinensis) during pregnancy.

Cherry Plum
Bach Flower Remedy

🏠 **Bach Flower Remedies® Ltd.**

⚗️ Contains: Prunus cerasifera 5x in 27% grape alcohol solution.

🤲 Take 2 drops under the tongue 4 times daily or 2 drops in a small glass of spring water and sip at intervals.

📦 10 ml with dropper.

🔢 Internal use.

💧 Liquid.

Chestnut Bud
Bach Flower Remedy

🏠 **Bach Flower Remedies® Ltd.**

Contains: Aesculus hippocas-tanum 5x in 27% grape alcohol solution.

Take 2 drops under the tongue 4 times daily or 2 drops in a small glass of spring water and sip at intervals.

10 ml with dropper.

Internal use.

Liquid.

Chewable Enzymes

Natural Factors® Nutritional Products Ltd.

Each tablet contains: Papain (from papaya fruit) 100 mg, Amylase 5 mg. Non-medicinal ingredient: Bromelain 15 mg.

Take 1 tablet at mealtime as an aid to digestion.

Available in 90 and 180 tablets.

Internal use. Contains no artificial preservatives, color, corn, dairy, gluten, soya, starch or yeast.

Tablet.

Visual.

Chewable Vitamin C

Albi Imports Ltd.

Each tablet contains: 500 mg of Vitamin C in a natural base.

Take 1–2 tablets daily or as

recommended by your health care professional.

Available in 90 tablets and varying strengths.

Internal use. Available in various strengths and three natural flavors: wildberry, orange juice and blackberry.

Powder.

Chewable tablet.

Chickweed

Nature's Herbs®

Each 389 mg capsule contains: Wild countryside® Chickweed herb.

Take 3 capsules 3 times daily with a large glass of water.

Available in 100 capsules.

Internal use. Preservative-free.

Capsule.

Chicory
Bach Flower Remedy

Bach Flower Remedies® Ltd.

Contains: Cichorium intybus 5x in 27% grape alcohol solution.

Take 2 drops under the tongue 4 times daily or 2 drops in a small glass of spring water and sip at intervals.

10 ml with dropper.

Internal use.

Liquid.

ChlorAid™
Internal Deodorant

Nature's Herbs®

Each capsule contains: Premium Chlorophyll concentrate (chlorophyll copper complex) 50 mg. Other ingredients include chlorophyll-rich green foods (highly digestible pure chlorella micro-algae, parsley herb, alfalfa leaves).

Take 1-2 capsules 2 times daily.
Children under 12 years of age; consult a doctor.

100 capsules.

Internal use.

Capsule.

If you are pregnant or nursing, seek the advice of a health professional before using this product.

Chondroitin Sulfate
500 mg

Natural Factors® Nutritional Products Ltd.

Each capsule contains: Chondroitin sulfate 500 mg, in a gelatin capsule with vegetable grade Magnesium stearate (used as a lubricant) and rice protein.

Take 2-3 capsules daily or as directed by a physician.

Available in 90 and 180 capsules.

Internal use. Contains no artificial preservatives, color, dairy, sweeteners, starch, wheat or yeast.

Capsule.

Visual.

Chromium GTF 500 mcg
Chelated

Natural Factors®
Nutritional Products Ltd.

Each tablet contains: elemental Chromium GTF (HVP* chelate) 500 mcg. *Hydrolyzed vegetable protein (sourced from rice).

Take 1 tablet daily or as directed by a physician.

Available in 90 tablets.

Internal use. Contains no artificial preservatives, color, dairy, sweeteners, starch, wheat or yeast.

Tablet.

Visual.

Cinnamon Leaf
Essential Oil

Bach-Karooch Ltd.

Contains: Cinnamomum zeylanicum 100%.

Two parts Essential oil must be diluted in 98 parts vegetable oil before applying to the skin. Consult Aromatherapy literature for specific methods of use and directions for each oil.

10 ml in amber bottle with child-resistant cap and one-drop insert.

Oil.

Possible skin irritant.

Caution: due to high concentration, all oils may be harmful if improperly used!
External use only.

Citronella
Essential Oil

Bach-Karooch Ltd.

Contains: Cymbopogen nardus 100%.

Two parts Essential oil must be diluted in 98 parts vegetable oil before applying to the skin. Consult Aromatherapy literature for specific methods of use and directions for each oil.

10 ml in amber bottle with child-resistant cap and one-drop insert.

Oil.

Possible dermatitis in some individuals.

Caution: due to high concentration, all oils may be harmful if improperly used!
External use only. Avoid during pregnancy.

Citrus Bioflavonoids
Plus Hesperidin

Natural Factors®
Nutritional Products Ltd.

Each 650 mg capsule contains: Bioflavonoid complex (lemon, orange, grapefruit) 500 mg,

Hesperidin 150 mg. Encapsulated in a gelatin capsule with vegetable grade Magnesium stearate (used as a lubricant).

Take 1-3 capsules daily.

Available in 90 capsules.

Internal use. Contains no artificial preservatives, color, dairy, sweeteners, starch, wheat or yeast.

Capsule.

Visual.

Citrus-Power®

Nature's Herbs®

Each capsule contains: 500 mg certified potency essential oil of orange, concentrated and standardized for a minimum of preferred 85% (425 mg) d-Limonene.

Take 1–2 capsules daily, preferably with a meal.

Available in 60 softgel capsules.

Internal use. Preservative-free.

Softgel capsule.

CL-7 Formula®

Nature's Herbs®

Each capsule contains: Mullein, Chickweed, Marshmallow root, Slippery elm bark, White pine bark, Elecampane root, and Hyssop.

Take 3 capsules 3 times daily with a large glass of water.

Available in 100 capsules.

Internal use. Preservative-free.

Capsule.

Clary Sage
Essential Oil

Bach-Karooch Ltd.

Contains: Salvia sclarea 100%.

Two parts Essential oil must be diluted in 98 parts vegetable oil before applying to the skin. Consult Aromatherapy literature for specific methods of use and directions for each oil.

10 ml in amber bottle with child-resistant cap and one-drop insert.

Oil.

Caution: due to high concentration, all oils may be harmful if improperly used!
External use only. Do not use when drinking alcohol; exaggerates drunken state. Avoid during pregnancy.

Clear Base™ E 400 iu

Natural Factors® Nutritional Products Ltd.

Each capsule contains: 400 IU, of a pure natural clear base. Vitamin E in the form of d-alpha Tocopheryl acetate, derived and isolated from 100% natural sources free from allergens.

Take 1-2 capsules daily or as directed by a physician.

Available in 60 and 90 capsules.

Internal use. Contains no artificial preservatives, color, dairy, soya, sweeteners, starch, wheat or yeast.

Softgel capsule.

Visual.

Clear Base™ E 800 iu

Natural Factors® Nutritional Products Ltd.

Each capsule contains: 800 IU, of pure natural clear base Vitamin E in the form of d-alpha Tocopheryl acetate, derived and isolated from 100% natural sources free from allergens.

Take 1 capsule daily or as directed by a physician.

Available in 60, 90 and 180 capsules.

Internal use. Contains no artificial preservatives, color, dairy, soya, sweeteners, starch, wheat or yeast.

Softgel capsule.

Visual.

Clematis
Bach Flower Remedy

Bach Flower Remedies® Ltd.

Contains: Clematis vitalba 5x in 27% grape alcohol solution.

Take 2 drops under the tongue 4 times daily or 2 drops in a small glass of spring water and sip at intervals.

10 ml with dropper.

Internal use

Liquid.

CLM

Nutra Research International

Contains: Beech, Vine, Rock rose, Impatiens, Star of Bethlehem, Vervain, Hops, Valerian, Amethyst water, 20% Ethanol USP.

Take 8 drops under the tongue 2-3 times daily on an empty stomach. Children: 4 drops.

Available in 1 oz.

Internal use. Hypoallergenic. Vegetarian.

Liquid sublingual.

Clove Bud
Essential Oil

Bach-Karooch Ltd.

Contains: Eugenia caryophyllata 100%.

Two parts Essential oil must be diluted in 98 parts vegetable oil before applying to the skin. Consult Aromatherapy literature for specific methods of use and directions for each oil.

10 ml in amber bottle with child-resistant cap and one-drop insert.

Oil.

Can cause skin and mucous membrane irritation; possible dermatitis in some individuals.

Caution: due to high concentration, all oils may be harmful if improperly used! External use only.

Co-Q-Max

CoEnzyme Q10 Plus Flax Oil

Flora Manufacturing & Distributing Ltd.

Each capsule contains: CoEnzyme Q10 (Ubiquinone) 30 mg, Flax oil (pressed from certified organically grown flax seed) 470 mg, in a gelatin capsule containing carob.

Take 1 or 2 capsules twice daily.

Available in amber bottle of 60 capsules.

Internal use.

Capsule.

Coenzyme Q10

30 mg

Natural Factors® Nutritional Products Ltd.

Each capsule contains: Coenzyme Q10 30 mg. Source of Ubiquinone.

Take 1-2 capsules daily or as directed by a physician.

Available in 30, 60 and 120 capsules.

Internal use. Contains no artificial preservatives, color, dairy, sweeteners, starch, wheat or yeast.

Capsule.

Visual.

Coenzyme Q10

60 mg

Natural Factors® Nutritional Products Ltd.

Each capsule contains: Coenzyme Q10 60 mg. Source of Ubiquinone.

Take 1-2 capsules daily or as directed by a physician.

Available in 30, 60 and 120 capsules.

Internal use. Contains no artificial preservatives, color, dairy, sweeteners, starch, wheat or yeast.

Capsule.

Visual.

Cold Control®

Nature's Herbs®

Each capsule contains: Power extract® 4:1 of Horehound 100 mg, Ephedra 4:1 50 mg, and Pseudoephedrine as naturally occurs in Certified Potency extract of Chinese ephedra herb 75 mg. Other ingredients: Natural herbs (Power extracts® of White willow bark 5:1, Licorice root 4:1, Chickweed, Mullein, Echinacea angustifolia, Parthenium integrifolium (Missouri snake root), Goldenseal root, Cayenne, Wild cherry bark and Rosehips).

Adults take 2-3 capsules every 4 hours up to 12 capsules daily. Children 6-12 take 1-2 capsules every 4 hours up to 6 capsules daily. Children under 6 use only as directed by a doctor.

Available in 60 capsules.

Internal use.

Capsule.

Individuals with high blood pressure, heart disease, diabetes, or thyroid disease should use only as directed by a doctor. If you are pregnant or nursing, seek the advice of a health professional before using this product. A persistent cough may be a sign of a serious condition. If cough persists for more than 1 week, tends to recur, or is accompanied by high fever, rash, or persistent headaches, consult a doctor. Do not take this product for persistent or chronic cough from smoking, asthma, or emphysema, if cough is accompanied by excessive mucus, or if you are presently taking a prescription anti hypertensive or antidepressant drug containing a Monoamine Oxidase (MOA) inhibitor unless directed by a doctor.

COLDENZA

Homeopathic Complex

A. Nelson & Company Ltd.

Each tablet contains: Anas barbariae hepatis et cordis extractum 6c, Arsenicum iodatum 6c, Gelsemium sempervirens 6c, Eupatorium perfoliatum 6c.

Take 2 tablets every hour for 6 doses, then 3 times daily until symptoms subside. Childen: half the adult dose.

72 tablets in blister packs.

Internal use.

Tablet.

Coltsfoot

W. Schoenenberger

Contains: Pure natural pressed herb and plant juice from organically grown Coltsfoot plants.

Shake bottle before use. Take 3 or 4 times daily before meals 1 tbsp. diluted in water, milk or tea, one part juice to six parts liquid. For children 1 tsp. full instead of tbsp. Unopened bottle will keep indefinitely: opened, for 6 days.

Amber bottle of 5.5 fl. oz.

Internal use. Organically grown in nearly ideal conditions in the Black Forest & Swabian uplands, where the air is pure the plants are gathered at the moment when their production of valuable ingredients is at its peak. The juices are extracted by specially designed hydraulic presses that ensure maximum recovery of all essential elements, making certain that not more than 2-3 hours elapse between harvesting, pressing and bottling.

Cellular plant juice.

Complete B 100 mg
Time Release

**Natural Factors®
Nutritional Products Ltd.**

Each tablet contains: Vitamin B-1 (Thiamine hydrochloride) 100 mg, Vitamin B-2 (Riboflavin) 100 mg, Niacinamide 100 mg, Vitamin B-6 (Pyridoxine hydrochloride) 100 mg, Vitamin B-12 (Cyanocobalamin) 100 mcg, Biotin 300 mcg, Folic acid 400 mcg, d-Pantothenic acid 100 mg. Lipotropic factors: Choline bitartrate 210 mg, Inositol 100 mg. Non-medicinal ingredient: Para Amino Benzoic acid 100 mg.

Take 1 tablet daily or as directed by a physician.

Available in 60, 90 and 180 tablets.

Internal use. Contains no artificial preservatives, color, corn, dairy, gluten, soya, starch, sweeteners or yeast.

Tablet.

Visual.

Complete Megazymes
Digestive Aid

**Natural Factors®
Nutritional Products Ltd.**

Each tablet contains: Amylase 50 mg, Betaine hydrochloride 50 mg, Bromelain 50 mg, Papain 25 mg, Papaya 6.5 mg. Non-medicinal ingredients: Fenugreek powder 50 mg, Okra 50 mg, Pectin 25 mg.

Take 1 tablet at mealtime.

Available in 90 and 180 tablets.

Internal use. Contains no artificial preservatives, color, dairy, sweeteners, starch, wheat or yeast.

Tablet.

Visual.

Complete Multi

**Natural Factors®
Nutritional Products Ltd.**

Each tablet contains: Vitamin A (Palmitate) 10,000 IU, Vitamin D3 400 IU, Vitamin B-1 (Thiamine hydrochloride) 10 mg, Vitamin B-2 (Riboflavin) 10 mg, Niacinamide 30 mg, Vitamin B-6 (Pyridoxine hydrochloride) 10 mg, Vitamin B-12 (Cyanocobalamin) 20 mcg, Pantothenic acid (Calcium pantothenate) 10 mg, Folic acid 0.2 mg, Biotin 10 mcg, Vitamin C (Ascorbic acid) 100 mg, Vitamin E (d-alpha Tocopheryl acetate) 25 IU, Lipotropic factors: Choline bitartrate 30 mg, Inositol 30 mg, Methionine 10 mg. Minerals: Calcium (citrate) 125 mg, Magnesium (oxide) 62.5 mg, Phosphorus (bone meal) 50 mg, Potassium (citrate) 10 mg, Iron (Ferrous fumerate) 8 mg, Manganese (citrate) 200 mcg, Iodine (kelp) 0.1 mg, Copper (gluconate) 0.1 mg. Non-medicinal ingredients: Para Amino Benzoic acid 10 mg, Citrus bioflavonoids 10 mg, Hesperidin 10 mg, Rutin 10 mg, Glutamic acid 10 mg, Alfalfa juice powder 10 mg, Lecithin 5 mg.

Take 1 tablet daily or as directed by a physician.

Available in 60, 90 and 180 tablets.

Internal use. Contains no artificial preservatives, color, dairy, sweeteners starch, wheat or yeast.

Tablet.

There is enough iron in this product to seriously harm a child.

Visual.

Cool B3

Niacin

Klaire Laboratories, Inc., USA & Europe

Each capsule contains: Niacin (Inositol hexanicotinate) 500 mg. Added ingredients: Cellulose and L-leucine. Inositol hexanicotinate is a non-flushing form of Niacin.

Take 1 capsule daily or as directed by a physician.

Available in 60 capsules.

Internal use. Non-flushing niacin eliminates the flushing side effects, gastrointestinal symptoms and toxicity problems.

Capsule.

Coreplex® Hawthorn Tonic

Flora Manufacturing & Distributing Ltd.

Each 500 ml bottle contains: Aqueous extracts of: Hawthorn blossoms and leaves (Crataegus oxyacantha), Passion flower herb (Passiflora incarnata), Hibiscus flowers (Hibiscus sabdariffa), Hawthorn berry extract (Crataegus sp.) (1:4) natural strawberry flavoring and Xanthan gum in a base of Purified water, Apple juice and Blackstrap molassses.

Take 3 to 4 tbsp. per day.

Available in 500 ml.

Internal use. Consume within 4 weeks of opening.

Tonic.

Pregnant and nursing women should consult a qualified health care practitioner before use.

Cough & Cold Formula

Natural Factors® Nutritional Products Ltd.

Each capsule contains: Ephedra extract (8% ephedrine) (Ephedra sinica) 100 mg, Ginger extract (4% volatile oil) (Zingiber officinale) 50 mg, Echinacea extract (0.7% flavonoids) (Echinacea purpurea) 25 mg, Goldenseal extract (5% hydrastine) (Hydrastis canadensis) 25 mg, Cool Capsicum powder (Capsicum frutescens) 50 mg, Wild cherry powder (Prunus serotina) 50 mg.

Take 1 to 3 capsules daily.

Available in 90 capsules.

Internal use. Contains no artificial preservatives, color, dairy, sweeteners, starch, wheat or yeast.

Capsule.

Do not exceed recommended dosage or take for more than 7 days except on the advice of a physician. Consult a physician prior to use if you have heart or thyroid disease, high blood pressure, diabetes, glaucoma, difficulty in urination due to prostate gland enlargement or are taking prescription drugs. Do not use if you currently take or have taken Monoamine Oxidase (MAO) inhibitor drugs. Do not consume during pregnancy.

Visual.

Crab Apple

Bach Flower Remedy

Bach Flower Remedies® Ltd.

Contains: Malus pumila 5x in 27% grape alcohol solution.

Take 2 drops under the tongue 4 times daily or 2 drops in a small glass of spring water and sip at intervals.

10 ml with dropper.

Internal use.

Liquid.

Cranberry Juice Concentrate

Nature's Herbs®

Each 505 mg capsule contains: Fresh whole dried Cranberry juice concentrate.

Take 2-4 capsules 3 times daily with a large glass of water preferably at mealtimes.

Available in 100 capsules.

Internal use. Preservative-free.

Capsule.

Cranberry Whole Fruit

Nature's Herbs®

Each 475 mg capsule contains: Cranberry whole fruit.

Take 2-4 capsules 3 times daily, preferably at mealtimes.

Available in 100 capsules.

Internal use. Preservative-free.

Capsule.

CS-Force™
Chondroitin Sulphate and Glucosamine Sulphate

Prairie Naturals®

Each capsule contains: Glucosamine sulfate (sodium-free) 300 mg, Chondroitin sulfate (70%) 240 mg, Bromelain pineapple enzyme (1600 mcu/g) 10 mg.

Take 1 capsule 3 times daily or as directed by a health professional.

Available in 90 and 180 capsules.

Internal use. Free of yeast, gluten, starch, soya, egg, dairy, artificial colors, preservatives, solvents or alcohol.

Capsule.

Visual.

Cuprum Met.
Homeopathic Remedy

A. Nelson & Company Ltd.

Each pillule contains: Cuprum metallicum 6c.

Take 2 pillules every 2 hours for the first 6 doses, then 4 times daily for up to 5 days. Pillules should be sucked or chewed and taken between meals.

84 pillules/globules per bottle.

Internal use.

Pillule/globule.

Curcumin-Power™

Nature's Herbs®

Each capsule contains: 300 mg certified potency Turmeric extract concentrated and standardized for a minimum of preferred 95% curcumins, in a synergistic base of whole Turmeric powder.

Take 1 capsule 2-3 times daily with a large glass of water.

Available in 60 capsules.

Internal use. Preservative-free.

Capsule.

Cypress
Essential Oil

Bach-Karooch Ltd.

Contains: Cupressus sempervirons 100%.

Two parts Essential oil must be diluted in 98 parts vegetable oil before applying to the skin. Consult Aromatherapy literature for specific methods of use and directions for each oil.

10 ml in amber bottle with child-resistant cap and one-drop insert.

Oil.

Caution: due to high concentration, all oils may be harmful if improperly used! External use only.

Daily Enzymes
Vegetarian

Nutra Research International

Each 500 mg capsule contains: Vegetal analog of Pancreatic protease 4X with acid stable Protease 300 mg, Lipase 125 mg, Alpha amylase 50 mg, Amyloglucosidase 13 mg, Cellulase 5 mg, Hemicellulase 3 mg, Lactase 5 mg.

Take 1 capsule with water at the beginning of each typical meal or sprinkle over food.

120 capsules.

Hypoallergenic. Broad spectrum blend of food enzymes.

Capsule.

Daily Supreme
MultiVitamin & Mineral

🏠 **Nutra Research International**

⚗️ Each tablet contains: Beta carotene (Provitamin A) 5000 IU, Vitamin B1 (Thiamine HCl) 25 mg, Vitamin B2 (Riboflavin) 25 mg, Vitamin B3 (Niacinamide) 25 mg, Vitamin B5 (Pantothenic acid) 25 mg, Vitamin B6 (Pyridoxin HCl) 25 mg, Vitamin B12 (Cyanocobalin) 50 mcg, Choline (bitartarate), Inositol 50 mg, PABA 15 mg, Biotin 50 mg, Folic acid 400 mcg, Vitamin C (Calcium ascorbate) 250 mg, Vitamin D (Calciferol) 100 IU, Vitamin E (d-alpha succinate) 100 IU, Minerals: Calcium (ascorbate, carbonate) 50 mg, Magnesium oxide (HVP*) 25 mg, Zinc (HVP* chelate) 7.5 mg, Iron (HVP* chelate) 5 mg, Potassium (HVP* chelate) 25 mg, Manganese (HVP* chelate) 2.5 mg, Selenium (HVP* chelate) 25 mcg, Chromium GTF 50 mcg, Iodine (kelp) 0.5 mg, Molybdenum (HVP* chelate) 25 mcg, Vanadium (HVP* chelate) 24 mcg, Copper (HVP* chelate) 0.5 mg. Non-medicinal ingredients: Spirulina, Chlorella 250 mg, Barley grass, Alfalfa juice 175 mg, 17 Amino acids 190 mg, Bee pollen, Ginseng 50 mg, Bioflavonoids, Rutin 38 mg, Psyllium, Echinacea 50 mg, Apple pectin, Betaine HCL 25 mg, Glutamic acid, Papain 25 mg, Pepsin, Lipase, Amylase 22.5 mg, Chlorophyll 4.5 mg. *Hydrolyzed vegetable protein.

📦 Available in 60 and 90 tablets.

 Internal use.

⊘ Tablet.

Damiana Leaves

🏠 **Nature's Herbs®**

⚗️ Each 384 mg capsule contains: Wild countryside® Damiana leaves.

🤝 Take 3-4 capsules 3 times daily with a large glass of water.

📦 Available in 100 capsules.

Ⅱ Internal use. Preservative-free.

▭ Capsule.

Dandelion Juice

🏠 **W. Schoenenberger**

⚗️ Contains: Pure natural pressed herb and plant juice from organically grown Dandelion plants.

🤝 Shake bottle before use. Take 3 or 4 times daily before meals 1 tbsp. diluted in water, milk or tea, one part juice to six parts liquid. For children 1 tsp. full instead of tbsp. Unopened bottle will keep indefinitely: opened, for 6 days.

📦 Amber bottle of 5.5 fl. oz.

Ⅱ Internal use. Organically grown in nearly ideal conditions in the Black Forest & Swabian uplands, where the air is pure. The plants are gathered at the moment when their production of valuable ingredients is at its peak. The juices are extracted by specially designed hydraulic presses that ensure maximum recovery of all essential elements, making certain that not more than 2-3 hours elapse between harvesting, pressing and bottling.

💧 Cellular plant juice.

Dandelion Root

🏠 **Nature's Herbs®**

⚗️ Each 515 mg capsule contains: Wild countryside® Dandelion root.

🤝 Take 3 capsules 3 times daily with a large glass of water.

📦 Available in 100 capsules.

Ⅱ Internal use. Preservative-free.

▭ Capsule.

Dandelion-Golden Seal Herbal Formula

🏠 **Nature's Herbs®**

⚗️ Each capsule contains: Dandelion root, Red beet root, Artichoke, Bayberry bark, Barberry bark, Yellow dock root, Goldenseal root, Turmeric extract (standardized at 95% curcumin), Milk thistle extract (standardized at 80% silymarin).

🤝 Take 2 capsules 3 times daily with a large glass of water.

📦 Available in 100 capsules.

Ⅱ Internal use. Preservative-free capsules.

▭ Capsule.

Dang Quei

Albi Imports Ltd.

Each capsule contains: 518 mg of pure Dang quei root powder.

Take 2 capsules 3 times daily.

Available in 50, 100 and 200 capsules.

Internal use.

Capsule.

Do not use during pregnancy.

DDS Acidophilus®

UAS Labs

Contains: Freeze dried Lactobacillus acidophilus (DDS strain), Fructooligosaccharides in a rice starch base. Contains 2 billion CFU/9m.

Take 2 capsules daily on an empty stomach.

Available in 100 capsules (bottle) or 2.5 oz. of powder.

Internal and external use. Non-dairy. Different formulations available for children and lactating mothers.

Capsule.

Powder.

Visual.

Derma-Force™

Prairie Naturals®

Each capsule contains: Vitamin C 117 mg, Vitamin A (Beta carotene) 3333.3 IU, Vitamin D3 100 IU, Vitamin B1 (Thiamine) 10 mg, Vitamin B2 (Riboflavin) 10 mg, Vitamin B3 (Niacinamide) 7 mg, Vitamin B6 (Pyridoxine HCL) 10 mg, Pantothenic acid 33.3 mg, Vitamin B12 33.3 mg, Vitamin E (d-alpha Tocopheryl succinate) 33.3 IU, Folic acid .333 mg, Biotin 300 mcg. Lipotropic factors: Choline (bitartrate) 25 mg, Inositol 25 mg, L-Methionine 25 mg. Minerals: Sulphur (naturally occurring from sulphur-containing amino acids) 8.33 mg, Calcium (citrate) 42 mg, Magnesium (citrate) 17 mg, Zinc (citrate) 8.33 mg. Non-medicinal ingredients: Lecithin 30 mg, Citrus bioflavonoids 25 mg, PABA 33.3 mg, L-Cysteine 25 mg. Organic herbal base: Curcumin turmeric (Curcuma longa) 25 mg, Burdock root (Arctium lappa) 25 mg, Aqueous extract of spring Horsetail (vegetal silica) 25 mg, Norwegian Kelp (Laminaria) 15 mg, Oat straw (Avena sativa) 25 mg.

Take 1-3 capsules daily or as directed by a physician.

Available in 90 and 180 capsules.

Internal use. Contains no yeast, gluten, egg, dairy, artificial color, preservatives, solvents or alcohol.

Capsule.

Visual.

Devil's Claw Extract

Nature's Herbs®

Contains: EuroQuality® extract of Devil's claw, standardized for 1% harpagoside, 6 g, in pure alpine spring water. Pure grain alcohol, 20% by volume.

Take 10-30 drops 3 times daily with water or juice. Shake well before use.

Available in 1 oz (30 ml).

Internal use.

Tincture.

Devil's Claw Extract 5:1

Prairie Naturals®

Each capsule contains: Devil's claw extract (Harpogophytum procumbens) 300 mg, Siberian ginseng (Eleuterococcus senticosus) 200 mg, (devil's claw secondary root extract 5:1, equivalent to 1500 mg devil's claw herb powder).

Take 1 capsule 3 times daily before meals.

Available in 90 capsules.

Internal use. Certified free of yeast, gluten, starch, soya, egg, dairy, artificial colors or preservatives.

Capsule.

Visual.

Devil's Claw Soothing Rub

Flora Herbal Cream

🏠 **Flora Manufacturing & Distributing Ltd.**

⚗️ Contains: Distilled water, certified organic unrefined Flax oil, glyceryl-stearate*, emulsifying wax*, Devil's claw extract, glycerine, glucose moisturizer, Camomile extract, Comfrey extract, Arnica extract, Menthol, Phenonip (cosmetic preservative), oil of Rosemary, Vitamin E. *Naturally derived from coconut.

🤲 Gently massage into affected areas, as required.

📦 60 and 120 ml in opaque jar.

🔲 External use only.

⚗️ Cream.

DHEA

🏠 **Scandinavian Natural Health & Beauty Products, Inc.**

⚗️ Each capsule contains: Dehydroepiandrosterone 25 or 50 mg. Excipients: Microcrystalline cellulose, Dicalcium phosphate, Magnesium stearate.

🤲 Take 25-50 mg daily or according to doctor's prescription.

📦 Available in 60 capsules of 25 mg and 50 mg dosages.

🔲 Internal use. Pharmaceutical grade DHEA.

💊 Capsule.

 High doses of DHEA may cause acne and unwanted hair growth in women, reversible with decreased intake.

Diabetiks™

🏠 **The Green Turtle Bay® Vitamin Co., Inc.**

⚗️ Each 2 tablets contains: Vitamins: A (as Beta-carotene) 500 IU, C (as Niacorbate) 150 mg, E 50 IU, B1 (as Thiamine) 20 mg, B2 (as Riboflavin) 2.5 mg, Niacin (as Niacinamide) 15 mg, B6 (as Pyridoxine) 12.5 mg, Folate (as Folic acid) 150 mcg, B12 (as Cyanocobalamin) 45 mcg, Biotin 125 mcg. Minerals: Magnesium (as glycinate) 150 mg, Zinc (as monomethionine) 7.5 mg, Selenium (as methionate) 17.5 mcg, Copper (chelate) 0.75 mg, Manganese (chelate) 2.5 mg, Chromium (as nicotinate) 150 mcg, Molybdenum (as sodium molybdate) 12.5 mcg. Bioflavonoids: Bilberry extract (25% anthocyanidin) 50 mg, Citrus bioflavonoids 12.5 mg, Gingko biloba (24% flavoglycosides) 10 mg, Green tea extract (catachins >8%) 20 mg, Huckleberry leaf 100 mg, Pine bark Extract-OPC-85% (procyanidin) 1 mg. Amino acids: L-Carnitine-L-Tartrate 7.5 mg, N-Acetyl-L-Cysteine (Glutathione precursor) 50 mg, Taurine 375 mg. Other: Coenzyme Q10 1 mg, Lipoic acid 5 mg.

🤲 Take 2 tablets twice daily in conjunction with a multi-vitamin at meal times.

📦 Available in bottles of 60 and 120 tablets.

🔲 Internal use.

⊘ Tablet.

Diar-Ease®

🏠 **Nature's Herbs®**

⚗️ Each capsule contains: Certified potency Activated charcoal 90 mg, Kaolin 90 mg, and Apple pectin 80 mg. Other ingredients: Soothing natural herbs (Agrimony, Power extract® of chamomile flowers 4:1, peppermint and anise seed.

🤲 Adults: 2-4 capsules at the first sign of diarrhea and after each bowel movement or as needed. Do not exceed 8 doses daily. Children 3 to under 12 years of age 1/4 adult dosage.

📦 Available in 60 capsules.

🔲 Internal use.

💊 Capsule.

⚠️ Unless directed by a doctor, do not use for more than 2 days or in the presence of fever, or in children under 3 years of age. If you are pregnant or nursing, seek the advice of a health professional before using this product.

Digestion Forte

🏠 **NaturPharm Inc.**

⚗️ Each capsule contains: Protease I 10,500 USP, Protease II 6,750 PC, Protease III 2,500 HUT, Protease IV 92.5 HUT. Amylase/ Gluco amylase 16,500 USP, Lipase II 100 LU, Lactase I 420 LacU, Sucrase/ Invertase 16 IA, Maltase/Malt Diastase 220

DP, Cellulose 1 450 CMC-aseU. All active through the pH range of 2-12.

Take 2 capsules with each meal.

Available in 90 and 180 capsules.

Internal use. Extra strength pure plant digestive enzyme formula.

Capsule.

Diuretic Formula

Natural Factors® Nutritional Products Ltd.

Each capsule contains: Uva-Ursi extract (10% arbutin) (Arctostaphylos Uva-Ursi) 100 mg, Dandelion leaf 4:1 extract (Taraxacum officinale) 50 mg, Juniper berry 4:1 extract (2% volatile oil) (Juniperus communis) 25 mg, Cranberry 18:1 extract (Vaccinium macrocarpum) 25 mg, Parsley root powder (Carum petroselinum) 100 mg, in a gelatin capsule with rice protein.

Take 1-3 capsules daily.

Available in 90 capsules.

Internal use. Contains no artificial preservatives, color, dairy, sweeteners, starch, wheat or yeast.

Capsule.

Do not consume Uva-Ursi during pregnancy.

Visual.

Diurtab®

Nature's Herbs®

Each tablet contains: 11 natural herbs: Certified potency extract of Uva ursi 20 mg, Uva ursi herb powder 120 mg, Shavegrass (horsetail) 120 mg, Power-Extract® 2:1 of Juniper berries 36 mg, Juniper berries powder 50 mg, Cornsilk 50 mg, Parsley 33 mg, Queen-of-the-Meadow 20 mg, Buchu leaves 20 mg, Goldenrod 15 mg, Cubeb berries 10 mg, with powdered cranberries and watermelon seed.

Adults take 2-3 tablets with meals, up to 12 tablets daily while symptoms persist.

Available in 60 tablets.

Internal use.

Tablet.

If you are pregnant or nursing, seek the advice of a health professional before using this product.

Dong Quai Power™

Nature's Herbs®

Each capsule contains: Certified potency Dong quai root extract 150 mg, (equivalent to 375-500 mg, of whole root), concentrated and standardized for a minimum of preferred .8-1.1% ligustilide (active component) in a synergistic base of Wild countryside® Dong quai root, gelatin.

Take 2 capsules with both morning and evening meals.

Available in 60 capsules.

Internal use.

Capsule.

Do not consume Dong quai (Angelica sinensis) during pregnancy.

Dong Quai Root

Nature's Herbs®

Each 535 mg capsule contains: Wild countryside® Chinese Dong quai root.

Take 3 capsules 3 times daily with a large glass of water.

Available in 100 capsules.

Internal use. Preservative-free.

Capsule.

Drosera
Homeopathic Remedy

A. Nelson & Company Ltd.

Each pillule contains: Drosera rotundifolia 6c.

Take 2 pillules every 2 hours for the first 6 doses, then 4 times daily for up to 5 days. Pillules should be sucked or chewed and taken between meals.

84 pillules/globules per bottle.

Internal use.

Pillule/globule.

E 400 iu Plus Selenium 100 mcg

🏠 **Natural Factors®
Nutritional Products Ltd.**

⚗️ Each tablet contains: Vitamin E 400 IU (d-alpha Tocopheryl succinate), Selenium (yeast) 100 mcg, Vitamin C 100 mg, Manganese (gluconate) 10 mg.

👐 Take 1-2 tablets daily or as directed by a physician.

📦 Available in 60 and 90 tablets.

🔠 Internal use. Contains no artificial preservatives, color, dairy, sweeteners, starch or wheat.

⊘ Tablet.

📷 Visual.

E+Magnesium with Hawthorn

🏠 **Dr. Dunner AG**

⚗️ Each capsule contains: Medicinal ingredients: Vitamin E (d-alpha tocopheryl acetate) 200 IU, Magnesium (from amino acid chelate) 24 mg. Non-medicinal ingredients: Hawthorn extract standardized 50 mg (derived from 75 mg leaves, 75 mg flowers, 50 mg fruits).

👐 Unless otherwise directed, take 2 capsules daily as a supplement, preferably before breakfast or lunch.

📦 Available in amber bottle 45, 90 and 180 capsules.

🔠 Internal use.

💊 Capsule.

E Plus High C
Natural Roll-On Deodorant

🏠 **Aubrey Organics®**

⚗️ Contains: Rosewater, Fatty acid base (Vitamin F cream) Aloe vera gel, natural grain alcohol, Calendula blossom oil, Vitamin E (d-alpha tocopherol), Calamine oil, Arnica blossom oil, Camomile oil, Vitamin C (citrus) and mixed wild-flower oils.

👐 Shake well before using. Apply to dry underarms. May be applied again if needed.

📦 Available in 3 fl. oz.

🔠 External use only. Vegan.

ECHINACEA

🏠 **naka Sales Ltd.**

⚗️ Contains: 1:1 Echinacea tincture from Echinacea purpurea root and angustifolia root. Contains 30% grain alcohol.

👐 Take 20-30 drops in a small amount of water 3-5 times daily before meals.

📦 Available in 50 ml.

🔠 Tincture made from fresh certified organic living herbs.

💧 Tincture.

Echinacea Angustifolia Extract

🏠 **Nature's Herbs®**

⚗️ Contains: EuroQuality® extract of Echinacea, standardized for 1% echinacosides, 6 g, in pure alpine spring water. Pure grain alcohol, 20% by volume.

👐 Take 10-30 drops 3 times daily with water or juice. Shake well before use.

📦 Available in 1 oz (30 ml).

🔠 Internal use.

💧 Tincture.

Echinacea Cold Formula

🏠 **Natural Factors®
Nutritional Products Ltd.**

⚗️ Each capsule contains: Echinacea purpurea extract 1:5 (.7% flavonoids) 100 mg, Ginger extract 1:8 (zingiber officinale) 4% Volatile oil 50 mg, Elderberry extract (Sambucus nigra) 50 mg, Astragalus root (Astragalus membranaceus) 50 mg, Wild cherry powder (Prunus virginiana) 50 mg, Goldenseal extract 1:6 (5% Hydrastine) 25 mg, in a gelatin capsule with vegetable grade Magnesium stearate (used as a lubricant).

👐 Take 1-3 capsules daily.

📦 Available in 90 capsules.

🔠 Internal use. Contains no artificial preservatives, color, dairy, sweeteners, starch, wheat or yeast.

Capsule.

Visual.

Echinacea Cough & Cold Formula

Natural Factors®
Nutritional Products Ltd.

Each capsule contains: Echinacea purpurea extract (0.7% flavonoids) 100 mg, Ephedra extract (Ma huang) (8% ephedrine) 100 mg, Ginger extract 1:8 (4% volatile oil) 50 mg, Wild cherry powder (Prunus virginiana) 50 mg, Goldenseal extract 1:6 (5% hydrastine) 25 mg.

Take 1-3 capsules daily.

Available in 30 and 90 capsules.

Internal use. Contains no artificial preservatives, color, dairy, sweeteners, starch, wheat or yeast.

Capsule.

Do not exceed recommended dosage or take for more than 7 days except on the advice of a physician. Consult a physician prior to use if you have heart or thyroid diseases, high blood pressure, diabetes, glaucoma, difficulty in urination due to prostate gland enlargement or are taking prescription drugs. Do not use if you currently take or have taken Monoamine Oxidase (MAO) inhibitor drugs.

Visual.

Echinacea Fresh Herb Tincture
Certified Organic

Natural Factors®
Nutritional Products Ltd.

Each ml (1 ml = 30 drops) contains: Echinacea flower and root (Echinacea purpurea), 100% pure grain alcohol.

Take 20 drops 3 times daily or 10 drops each half hour in a glass of water.

Available in 30, 50 and 100 ml.

Internal use. All herbs in this product are certified organic or transitional (transitional means in the process of being certified).

Tincture.

Visual.

Echinacea Golden Seal Herbal Formula

Nature's Herbs®

Each capsule contains: Echinacea angustifolia root, Parthenium root, Goldenseal root, Burdock root, Dandelion root, and Cayenne.

Take 2-3 capsules 3 times daily with water, or unsweetened apple or cranberry juice.

Available in 100 capsules.

internal use. Preservative-free.

Capsule.

Echinacea & Goldenseal
Fresh Herb Tincture

Natural Factors®
Nutritional Products Ltd.

Each ml (1 ml = 30 drops) contains: Echinacea flower & root (Echinacea purpurea) & Goldenseal root in a 3:1 ratio. 100% pure grain alcohol.

Take 20 drops 3 times daily or 10 drops each half hour in a glass of water.

Available in 50 ml.

Internal use. All herbs in this product are certified organic or transitional (transitional means in the process of being certified). Fresh herb tincture.

Tincture.

Visual.

Echinacea Juice

W. Schoenenberger

Contains: Pure natural pressed herb-and plant juice from organically grown Echinacea plants.

Shake bottle before use. Take 3 or 4 times daily before meals 1 tbsp. diluted in water, milk or tea, one part juice to six parts liquid. For children 1 tsp. instead of tbsp. Unopened bottle will keep indefinitely: opened, for 6 days.

Amber bottle of 5.5 fl. oz.

Internal use. Organically grown in nearly ideal conditions in the Black Forest & Swabian uplands, where the air is pure. The plants are gathered at the moment when their production of valuable ingredients is at its peak. The juices are extracted by specially designed hydraulic presses that ensure maximum recovery of all essential elements, making certain that not more than 2-3 hours elapse between harvesting, pressing and bottling.

○ Cellular plant juice.

Echinacea Liquid Extract
Alcohol Free
Berry Flavor

⌂ **Natural Factors®
Nutritional Products Ltd.**

⚗ Contains: Echinacea flower and root extract (Echinacea purpurea), pure concentrate of fruit (berries) in a base of glycerin.

✍ Take 20 drops 3 times daily or 10 drops each half hour in a glass of water.

⧉ Available in 30 and 50 ml.

Ⓘ Internal use. All herbs in this product are certified organic or transitional (transitional means in the process of being certified).

⚲ Tincture.

📷 Visual.

Echinacea Power®

⌂ **Nature's Herbs®**

⚗ Each capsule contains: 125 mg Certified potency Echinacea

angustifolia root extract concentrated and standardized for a minimum of preferred 3.2-4.8% echinacoside, in a base of Wild countryside® Parthenium root, Echinacea angustifolia root and Echinacea purpurea root.

✍ Take 2 capsules 2-3 times daily with water.

⧉ Available in 60 capsules.

Ⓘ Internal use. Preservative-free. Two capsules are equivalent to five capsules of unconcentrated Echinacea.

 Capsule.

Echinacea Throat Spray
with Bee Propolis

⌂ **Natural Factors®
Nutritional Products Ltd.**

⚗ Contains: Echinacea, Licorice root, Forsythia fruit, Slippery elm bark, Cloves, Propolis, Myrrh and Goldenseal root in a base of approx. 20% grain alcohol, vegetable glycerin and Black cherry flavor. Contains standardized Echinacea and Bee Propolis extracts.

✍ Spray 2-3 times in mouth as needed for sore throat and gum pain, for lubricating dry mouth and throat and also as a breath freshener.

⧉ Available in 30 ml.

Ⓘ Internal use.

○ Spray bottle.

📷 Visual.

Echinacea Tincture
Triple Strength

⌂ **Natural Factors®
Nutritional Products Ltd.**

⚗ Each ml (1 ml = 30 drops) contains: Echinacea purpurea. Concentrated to 3 times the potency by a special fluid extraction process. 100% pure grain alcohol.

✍ Take 7 drops 3 times daily or 4 drops each half hour in a glass of water.

⧉ Available in 30 and 50 ml.

Ⓘ Internal use. All herbs in this product are certified organic or transitional (transitional means in the process of being certified).

⚲ Tincture.

📷 Visual.

Echinacea Tincture

⌂ **Salus-Haus**

⚗ Each 10 g tincture contains: 10 g extract derived from 1.5 g Echinacea root-radix Echinacea.

✍ Unless otherwise directed, take 15-30 drops diluted in a small amount of liquid 3 times daily.

⧉ Available in 50 ml, includes a dropper.

Ⓘ Internal use. Salus herbal tinctures are made in accordance with strictest health food principles, using natural ingredients only.

Tincture.

Visual.

Echinaforce®
A. Vogel
Echinacea Purpurea Tincture

Bioforce AG

Contains: Fresh organically grown Echinacea purpurea herb mother tincture 0.95 ml, fresh organically grown Echinacea purpurea root mother tincture 0.05 ml.

Take 20-30 drops, 3-5 times daily, in a small amount of water. Salivate before swallowing.

Available in 50 ml and 100 ml; and 120 tablets.

Internal use. Organic.

Tincture.

Tingling effect normal - due to Echinacea root extract.

Not for individuals suffering from leukemia unless otherwise prescribed by a physician. Should not be used in cases of multiple sclerosis and auto-immune disorders. Should not be administered to patients with a known allergy to plants of the compositae family.

Echinamide™ Cough Syrup
Alcohol Free

Natural Factors® Nutritional Products Ltd.

Each tsp. contains: Echinacea purpurea extract 1.2:1 (high in polysaccharides) 975 mg,

Mullein leaf extract 1.2:1 (Verbascum thapsus) 530 mg, Wild cherry bark extract 2.5:1 (Prunus Virginiana) 445 mg, Echinacea purpurea extract 4.2:1 (high in amides) 260 mg, Peppermint leaf extract 2.75:1 (Mentha piperita) 220 mg, Horehound leaf extract 1.77:1 (Marrubium vulgare) 110 mg, Menthol oil 3 mg, Eucalyptus oil (Eucalyptus globulus) 2.6 mg, Peppermint oil (Mentha Piperita) 1.6 mg. Non-medicinal ingredient: Lemon oil 8.5 mg. Echinacea honey (from hives in the Echinacea fields of Factor Farms) and glycerin. Made from fresh and standardized herb extracts.

Take 1-6 tsp. daily or as directed by a physician.

Available in 150 ml.

Contains no artificial preservatives, color, corn, dairy, gluten, soya, starch or yeast.

Syrup.

If cough persists for more than 7 days discontinue use and consult a physician.

Visual.

Efalex® Focus
Essential Fatty Acid and Vitamin E Supplement

Efamol Research Institute

Each 425 mg capsule contains: Medicinal: Cis-linoleic acid (from Evening primrose oil) 108 mg, Gamma-linolenic acid (from Evening primrose oil) 13.5 mg, Vitamin E (as dl-alpha Tocopheryl acetate) 20 IU. Non-medicinal: Tuna oil 260 mg, Thyme oil 3 mg.

Take 2 capsules twice daily.

Available in 90 capsules.

Internal use.

Capsule.

Efamol® Evening Primrose Oil

Efamol Research Institute

Each capsule contains (approximate composition): Evening primrose oil 500 mg, Cis-linoleic acid (LA from Evening primrose oil) 72%, Gamma-linolenic acid (GLA from Evening primrose oil) 9%, Oleic acid (OA from Evening primrose oil) 10%, other fatty acids (from Evening primrose oil) 9%, Vitamin E (as d-alpha Tocopheryl acetate) 13.6 IU.

Adults: Take 2 capsules 2 to 4 times daily, or as directed by a physician.
Children over 5 years: Give one half the adult dosage.

Available in amber bottle 90 and 180 capsules.

Internal use.

Capsule.

Side effects are rare and may be evidenced as stool softening, a normal response to ingestion of any oil; nausea, if taken on an empty stomach; or headache in individuals susceptible to alcohol-induced migraine.

Visual.

Efamol® Extra Strength Pure Evening Primrose Oil

Efamol Research Institute

Each capsule contains: Medicinal: Evening primrose oil 1000 mg, Cis-linoleic acid (LA from Evening primrose oil) 729 mg, Gamma-linolenic acid (GLA from Evening primrose oil) 90 mg, Vitamin E (as dl-alpha Tocopheryl acetate) 27 IU.

Take 1-2 capsules twice daily.

Available in amber bottle 120 capsules.

Internal use.

Capsule.

Side effects are rare and may be evidenced as stool softening, a normal response to ingestion of any oil; nausea, if taken on an empty stomach; or headache in individuals susceptible to alcohol-induced migraine.

Efamol® Fortify
Calcium, Essential Fatty Acid and Vitamin E Supplement

Efamol Research Institute

Each 750 mg capsule contains: Evening primrose oil with Calcium and non-medicinal fish oil. Medicinal: Cis-linoleic acid (LA from Evening primrose oil) 255 mg, Gamma-linolenic acid (GLA from Evening primrose oil) 30 mg, Calcium (as Calcium carbonate) 100 mg, Vitamin E (as d-alpha Tocopheryl acetate) 13.6 IU. Non-medicinal : Fish oil 44 mg.

Take 1 or 2 capsules twice daily with liquid at mealtimes, or as directed by a physician.

Available in amber bottle 90 capsules.

Internal use.

Capsule.

Efamol® Pure Liquid Evening Primrose Oil

Efamol Research Institute

Each ml contains: Medicinal: Evening primrose oil 930 mg, Cis-linoleic acid (72%, from Evening primrose oil), 670 mg, Gamma-linolenic acid (9%, from Evening primrose oil) 84 mg. Non-medicinal: Ronoxan A 1.8 mg.

Take 1/4 tsp. (25 drops) twice daily with food. Use within one month after opening or within 3 months if stored in a refrigerator.

Available in 30 ml.

Internal use. Easy to use dropper bottle for accurate measuring, suitable for vegetarians and ideal for those who find capsules difficult to swallow.

Oil.

Elderberry Flowers and Berries

Nature's Herbs®

Each 485 mg capsule contains: Powdered Elderberry flowers & berries.

Take 2-3 capsules 2-3 times daily with water.

Available in 100 capsules.

Internal use. Preservative-free.

Capsule.

Elm
Bach Flower Remedy

Bach Flower Remedies® Ltd.

Contains: Ulmus procera 5x in 27% grape alcohol solution.

Take 2 drops under the tongue 4 times daily or 2 drops in a small glass of spring water and sip at intervals.

10 ml with dropper.

Internal use.

Liquid.

Enriching Greens®
with Phytosomes™

Natural Factors® Nutritional Products Ltd.

3 tsp. contain a blend of: Alfalfa, Barley and Wheat Grass Juice Powder (Certified Organic) 3179 mg, Pure Soya Lecithin (99% oil free, 96% phosphatides) 1490 mg, Carrot Juice Powder (Organic) 680 mg, Phosphatidyl Choline 543 mg, Hawaiian Spirulina Pacifica (Organic) 425 mg, Apple Pectin Powder 425 mg, Phosphatidyl Inositol 330 mg, CGF Chlorella (Broken Cell Wall) 255 mg. Non-dairy probiotic culture: rhamnosus, aci-

dophilus in a base of FOS 200 mg, Peace River Bee Pollen powder 200 mg, Stevia 101 mg, Freeze-dried Mango 100 mg, Black Currant 5 mg. Standardized Extracts: Dandelion Root Extract 4:1 128 mg, Beetroot Extract (3% Betanin) 120 mg, Siberian Ginseng Extract 0.4% 85 mg, Pacific Kelp 4:1 Extract (Certified Purity) 85 mg, Artichoke 4:1 Extract 2% 40 mg, Soya Extract (25% Saponins, 10% isoflavone glycosides) 17 mg, Bilberry Extract 5:1 10 mg, Pineapple Extract (Bromelain 1000GDU) 5 mg, Cranberry Juice Extract 18:1 5 mg, Rosehip Extract 4:1 4 mg, Lycopene 3 mg. Phytosome™ Complex: Milk Thistle Phytosome™ 50 mg, Ginkgo Biloba Phytosome™ 10 mg, Grape Seed Phytosome™ 5 mg.

Shake or stir 3 tsp. of powder in 1 cup of juice or water. For a meal in a glass, blend with 1 cup of apple juice, 1/2 banana, and ice to cool.

Available in 150 or 300 g.

Powder.

Do not use this product if allergic to pollen.

Visual.

Epresat Herbal Multivitamin

Salus-Haus

Each measuring capful (22 g) contains: Medicinal ingredients: Vitamin A 10,000 IU, Vitamin D3 400 IU, Vitamin C 150 mg, Niacinamide 45 mg, Vitamin E 25 IU, Riboflavin 5.5 mg, Thiamine

4.5 mg. Pyridoxine hydrochloride 3 mg. Herbal ingredients: 9.56 g Hydrous liquid herb extract from: Blessed thistle 180 mg, Kola seeds 162 mg, Brown algae 135 mg, Wheat germ 45 mg, Echinacea 18 mg. In a base of: 6.20 g fruit juice concentrate (orange juice, passion fruit juice, guava juice, apricot nectar), 2 g hydrous yeast extract equivalent to 2.52 g dried yeast; 3.6 g fructose syrup equivalent to 2.52 g fruit sugar.

Take 1 measuring capful daily before a meal. May be mixed with fruit juices.

Available in bottles of 10 ml trial size, 250 and 500 ml

Internal use.

Liquid multivitamin supplement.

Visual.

Essiac® Herbal Formula

Essiac® International

Contains: Burdock root, Sheep sorrel, Slippery elm, Indian rhubarb root.

Take 2 oz. every 12 hours.

Available in 42.5 g.

Internal and external use. Organic.

Herbal Tea.

Powder.

Visual.

Ester-C®
600 mg Plus Bioflavonoids

Natural Factors® Nutritional Products Ltd.

Each capsule contains: Vitamin C 600 mg, elemental Calcium 80 mg. Non-medicinal ingredients: Bioflavonoids 100 mg, in a base of Rosehips, Hesperidin and Quercetin.

Take 1-2 capsules daily or as directed by a physicians.

Available in 60, 90 and 180 capsules.

Internal use. Contains no artificial preservatives color, dairy, sweeteners starch, wheat or yeast. pH neutral and buffered with Calcium.

Capsule.

Visual.

Ester-C® Calcium Ascorbate

Inter-Cal Corporation

Contains: Vitamin C, C metabolites and Calcium in the form of a patented calcium ascorbate.

Take as needed or as recommended by your health care practitioner.

Various potencies available.

Internal and external use. Ester-C® calcium ascorbate is a patented, non-acidic, Body-Ready® form of Vitamin C used in premium and advanced nutritional formulations and delivery system. Formulation, potency and packaging is determined by the individual companies.

Capsule.

Cream.

Liquid.

Powder.

Chewable tablet.

Because of its calcium content, Ester-C® ascorbate is contraindicated in hypercalcemic states, e. g., from dosing with parathyroid hormone, over dosage of Vitamin D, or dysfunctional calcium metabolism. High-dose supplementation with Vitamin C is contraindicated in individuals predisposed to form urinary calcium oxalate stones.

Eucalyptus
Essential Oil

Bach-Karooch Ltd.

Contains: Eucalyptus globulus 100%.

Two parts Essential oil must be diluted in 98 parts vegetable oil before applying to the skin. Consult Aromatherapy literature for specific methods of use and directions for each oil.

10 ml in amber bottle with child-resistant cap and one-drop insert.

Oil.

Caution: due to high concentration, all oils may be harmful if improperly used! External use only.

Eucalyptus (lemon)
Essential Oil

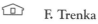

Bach-Karooch Ltd.

Contains: Eucalyptus citriodora 100%.

Two parts Essential oil must be diluted in 98 parts vegetable oil before applying to the skin. Consult Aromatherapy literature for specific methods of use and directions for each oil.

10 ml in amber bottle with child-resistant cap and one-drop insert.

Oil.

Possible skin irritant for some individuals.

Caution: due to high concentration, all oils may be harmful if improperly used! External use only.

Eucalyptus Spa Bath

Aubrey Organics®

Contains: Vegetable glycerine, Sweet almond oil, Seaware herb, Sea salts, Aloe vera, Ginger, Cinnamon, Vitamin F, Blue bottle, Camomile, St. John's wort, Marigold, Limetree, Rosemary, Sage, Witch hazel, Eucalyptus, Menthol, Ascorbic acid and Citrus seed extract.

Pour 1 capful into tub of hot water. Relax in tub and breathe in steam as it rises.

Available in 8 oz.

External use only. Can be used in vaporizer as well. All natur-

al herbal bath emulsion with eucalyptus. Vegan.

Bath emulsion.

Eucarbon®

F. Trenka

Each tablet contains: Medicinal ingredients: Senna leaf 105 mg, Sulphur 50 mg, Rhubarb powdered extract 1:1 25 mg. Non-medicinal ingredients: Non-activated vegetable source carbon 180 mg, Peppermint oil 0.5 mg, Fennel oil 0.5 mg.

Take 3-4 tablets may be taken daily or before bedtime.

Available in 30 tablets blister-packed and tins of 100.

Internal use.

Tablet.

Do not use in the presence of abdominal pain, nausea, fever or vomiting. Do not take for more than one week, unless under the advice of a physician. A laxative should not be taken within 2 hours of another medicine, because the desired effect of the other medicine may be reduced. For occasional use only.

Euphrasia
Homeopathic Remedy

A. Nelson & Company Ltd.

Each pillule contains: Euphrasia officinalis 6c.

Take 2 pillules every 2 hours for the first 6 doses, then 4 times daily for up to 5 days. Pillules should be sucked or chewed and taken between meals.

84 pillules/globules per bottle.

Internal use.

Pillule/globule.

Evening Primrose Complexion and Body Lotion

Aubrey Organics®

Contains: Aubrey's essential fatty acid base (Vitamin F, Aloe vera, Coconut fatty acid base), Vitaplant complex (Avocado oil, St. John's wort oil, Arnica oil, Wheat germ oil, Calendula oil, Aristolochia oil, Echinacea root oil), PABA, Evening primrose oil, Carrot oil, (Provitamin A, Pantothenate B5), Vitamin E, Lavender oil, Vitamin C, Citrus seed extract.

Apply a generous amount after bath or cleansing. Massage lotion in.

Available in 4 and 8 oz. bottles.

External use only.

Lotion.

Evergreen Wheatgrass Juice®

Evergreen Wheatgrass Juices Inc.

Contains: 100% Wheat grass juice.

Take 1 to 2 oz. daily. Due to its high enzyme content and totally predigested state it must be taken on a completely empty stomach, preferably in the morning. It can be diluted with water if desired. Wait 15 minutes before eating solid food. Because of it's oxygen content, avoid taking in the evening unless you want to stay awake.

Available in 10 oz. package, divided into 10 individual frozen portions.

Does not contain gluten, therefore safe for those with allergies to wheat. The young grass is in a vegetable state and safe to consume with all medications. Sun sweetened, tastes similar to watermelon.

Frozen liquid.

To preserve nutrients, do not mix with hot liquids.

Exsativa®

Scandinavian Natural Health & Beauty Products, Inc.

Each tablet contains: Avena sativa (Green oats) extract 300 mg, Nettle extract 150 mg, Sea buckthorn fruit extract 100 mg. Excipients: Microcrystalline cellulose, Dicalcium phosphate, Microcrystalline silicone dioxide, Hydrogenated soy bean oil.

Take 1-2 tablets daily as needed.

Available in blister packs of 30 per box.

Internal use.

Tablet.

Eye Formula

Natural Factors® Nutritional Products Ltd.

Each capsule contains: Eye bright 4:1 extract (Euphrasia officinalis) 100 mg, Bilberry 5:1 extract (Vaccinium myrtillus) 50 mg, Multi-Anthocyanidins (5% anthocyanidins) 15 mg, Carrot juice powder 25 mg, Rutin 25 mg, Quercetin 25 mg, in a gelatin capsule with rice protein.

Take 1-3 capsules daily.

Available in 90 capsules.

Internal use. Contains no artificial preservatives, color, dairy, sweeteners, starch, wheat or yeast.

Capsule.

Visual.

Eye Power™

Nature's Herbs®

Five capsules contain: Beta-carotene (Provitamin A) 50,000 IU, natural Vitamin E (succinate) 800 IU, Vitamin C 2000 mg, Zinc (from Zinc picolinate) 30 mg, Selenium (from selenomethionine) 200 mcg, Taurine 200 mg, N-acetyl cysteine 200 mg, L-glutathione

10 mg, Vitamin B2 50 mg, Chromium (from ChromeMate, Chromium nicotinate) 200 mcg, Certified potency Bilberry (Vaccinium myrtillus) extract (standardized for 25% anthocyanosides) 80 mg, Certified potency Ginkgo biloba extract (standardized for 24% flavonoid glycosides) 20 mg, Quercetin 250 mg.

Take 3-5 capsules daily with meals or as recommended by a health professional.

Available in 60 capsules.

Internal use.

Capsule.

Eyebright

Nature's Herbs®

Each 440 mg capsule contains: Wild countryside® Eyebright herb.

Take 1-2 capsules 3 times daily with a full glass of water.

Available in 100 capsules.

Internal use. Preservative-free.

Capsule.

Eyebright

Nature's Herbs®

Each 444 mg capsule contains Wild Countryside® Eyebright Herb.

Take 1-2 capsules 3 times daily with a large glass of water.

100 capsules.

Internal use. Preservative-free.

Capsule.

Feet Relief Massage Cream

Aubrey Organics®

Contains: Coconut fatty acid, Coconut fatty alcohol, organic Aloe vera fillet, Shea butter, White camellia oil, Peppermint oil, Menthol oil, Eucalyptus oil, Cayenne pepper oil (Capsicum), Camomile oil, Citrus seed extract and Vitamins A, E and C.

Apply a generous amount into palms and rub onto feet.

Available in 4 oz.

External use only. Vegan.

Cream.

Do not use on broken skin.

FemChange

Nature's Herbs®

Each 384 mg capsule contains: Pennyroyal herb, Blue cohosh root, Black cohosh root, Cramp bark, False unicorn root, Bayberry bark, Uva ursi leaf, Blessed thistle herb, Ginger root, Red raspberry leaves, Valerian root and Squawvine herb.

Take 3 capsules 3 times daily with a large glass of water.

100 capsules.

Internal use. Preservative-free.

Capsule.

Fennel

Essential Oil

Bach-Karooch Ltd.

Contains: Foeniculum vulgare 100%.

Two parts Essential oil must be diluted in 98 parts vegetable oil before applying to the skin. Consult Aromatherapy literature for specific methods of use and directions for each oil.

10 ml in amber bottle with child-resistant cap and one-drop insert.

Oil.

Caution: due to high concentration, all oils may be harmful if improperly used!
External use only. Avoid during pregnancy or if epileptic.

Fennel Seed

Nature's Herbs®

Each 455 mg capsule contains: Premium Fennel seed.

Take 2-3 capsules 3 times daily with a large glass of water.

Available in 100 capsules.

Internal use. Preservative-free.

Capsule.

Fenugreek Seed

🏠 **Nature's Herbs®**

⚗️ Each 626 mg capsule contains: Premium Fenugreek seed.

🖐️ Take 1 capsule 2-3 times daily with a large glass of water.

📦 Available in 100 capsules.

Ⅱ Internal use. Preservative-free.

💊 Capsule.

Fenugreek-Thyme Herbal Formula

🏠 **Nature's Herbs®**

⚗️ Each 505 mg capsule contains: Fenugreek seed and Thyme.

🖐️ Take 2 capsules 3 times daily with a large glass of water.

📦 Available in 100 capsules.

Ⅱ Internal use. Preservative-free.

💊 Capsule.

Ferrum Phos.
Homeopathic Remedy

🏠 **A. Nelson & Company Ltd.**

⚗️ Each pillule contains: Ferrum phosphoricum 6c.

🖐️ Take 2 pillules every 2 hours for the first 6 doses, then 4 times daily for up to 5 days. Pillules should be sucked or chewed and taken between meals.

📦 84 pillules/globules per bottle.

Ⅱ Internal use.

⊘ Pillule/globule.

Feverfew-Power®

🏠 **Nature's Herbs®**

⚗️ Each capsule contains: Certified potency Feverfew extract concentrated and standardized for a minimum of preferred 100 mcg sesquiterpene lactones, in a base of Vitamin E and vegetable oil.

🖐️ Take 1 capsule 3 times daily with a large glass of water.

📦 Available in 60 softgel capsules.

Ⅱ Internal use. Preservative-free.

💊 Softgel capsule.

⚠️ Do not use if you are pregnant or nursing.

Fir Needle
Essential Oil

🏠 **Bach-Karooch Ltd.**

⚗️ Contains: Abies siberica 100%.

🖐️ Two parts Essential oil must be diluted in 98 parts vegetable oil before applying to the skin. Consult Aromatherapy literature for specific methods of use and directions for each oil.

📦 10 ml in amber bottle with child-resistant cap and one-drop insert.

💧 Oil.

⚠️ Caution: due to high concentration, all oils may be harmful if improperly used! External use only.

Flax Oil
Linseed Oil

🏠 **Flora Manufacturing & Distributing Ltd.**

⚗️ Contains: Certified organically grown flax seeds.

🖐️ Use uncooked only (on salads, Budwig cream, etc.)

📦 Available in amber bottles of 250 and 500 ml.

Ⅱ Internal use. Organic. Flora flax oil is freshly pressed in an oxygen and light-free environment, at temperatures not exceeding 36 C (97 F). It is unrefined, non-deodorized, unfiltered and nitrogen flushed to preserve freshness. Once opened, best consumed within 3 weeks.

💧 Liquid.

⚠️ Do not heat flax oil.

📷 Visual.

Flax-O-Mega® Golden Flax Oil
1000 mg

🏠 **Flora Manufacturing & Distributing Ltd.**

⚗️ Each capsule contains: Flax seed oil (cold-pressed, certified organic) 1000 mg, Omega 3 (linolenic acid) 45-60%, Omega 6 (linoleic acid) 16-20%, Omega 9 (oleic acid) 16-22%.

Take 1 or 3 capsules up to 3 times daily.

Available in 90 and 180 capsules.

Internal use. Certified organic. The capsules do not require refrigeration. Flax-O-Mega® is made with 100% certified organic golden Flax seed oil, freshly cold-pressed in an oxygen and light-free environment at temperatures not exceeding 36 C (97 F). Unrefined, non-deodorized and unfiltered, in a gelatin capsule containing carob to protect against light.

Capsule.

Flaxseed Oil 1000 mg

Fresh Cold Pressed

Natural Factors® Nutritional Products Ltd.

Each capsule contains: Flaxseed oil, high lignan content (Linum usitatissimum) 1000 mg with d-alpha Tocopherol and gamma Tocopherol.

Take 1-3 capsules 3 times daily or as directed by a physician.

Available in 90, 180 and 360 capsules.

Internal use. Contains no artificial preservatives or color, corn, dairy, gluten, starch or yeast. *Lignans are natural phytochemicals found in high concentrations in flaxseeds.

Softgel capsule.

Visual.

Flor-Essence Herbal Tea Blend®

Liquid

Flora Manufacturing & Distributing Ltd.

Contains: Purified water, aqueous extracts of: Burdock root (Arctium lappa)*, Sheep sorrel herb (Rumex acetosella), Slippery elm bark (Ulmus rubra), Watercress herb (Nasturtium officinale), Turkish rhubarb root (Rheum palmatum), Kelp (Laminaria digitata), Blessed thistle herb (Carduus benedictus)*, Red clover blossom (Trifolium pratense)*.
*Certified Organic.

Take 1-2 oz., 1-2 times daily. Dilute with an equal or double amount of unfluoridated, purified, hot or cold water, and sip slowly.
Children: use 1/2 the recommended amount.
Important: take on an empty stomach, a.m. and p.m.

Available in 500 ml and dry herbs.

Internal use. Authorized by Elaine Alexander. Contains no caffeine, preservatives or artificial colors. Certified organic. Safe to take in conjunction with other therapies or medications.

Herbal extraction.

Visual.

Flor-Essence Herbal Tea Blend®

Dry Herbal Tea Blend

Flora Manufacturing & Distributing Ltd.

Contains: Burdock root (Arctium lappa)*, Sheep sorrel herb (Rumex acetosella), Slippery elm bark (Ulmus rubra), Watercress herb (Nasturtium officinale), Turkish rhubarb root (Rheum palmatum), Kelp (Laminaria digitata), Blessed thistle herb (Carduus benedictus)*, Red clover blossom (Trifolium pratense)*.
*Certified Organic.

Follow instructions on label.

Box contains 3 packets of 21 g of powdered herbs.

Internal use. Authorized by Elaine Alexander. Contains no caffeine, preservatives or artificial colors. Certified organic. Safe to take in conjunction with other therapies or medications.

Dry powdered herbs.

Flora-Vision® Bilberry Extract

Flora Manufacturing & Distributing Ltd.

Each vegetarian capsule contains: Standardized aqueous alcohol extract of bilberries (25% anthocyanins, 36% anthocyanosides) 1:100 250 mg, Freeze-dried blueberries (powdered) 100 mg.

Take 1 or 2 capsules twice daily with meals. For maximum absorption, take with berries, fruits or fruit juices.

Available in amber bottles of 30 and 60 capsules.

Internal use.

Vegicaps® (non-animal source, easily digested capsule).

Floradix® Floravit
Yeast-Free Iron and Vitamin Supplement

Salus-Haus

Each capful (20 ml) contains: Medicinal ingredients: Iron (II) from gluconate 19.1 mg, Vitamin C (Ascorbic acid) 21.2 mg, Vitamin B1 (Thiamine hydrochloride) 1.6 mg, Vitamin B2 (Riboflavin) 1.7 mg, Vitamin B6 (Pyridoxine hydrochloride) 1.7 mg, Vitamin B12 (Cyanocobalamine) 2.0 mcg; in a non-medical base of juices: grape, pear, blackcurrant, cherry, blackberry and carrot; and aqueous herbal extracts of: Rosehips, African mallow blossoms, Camomile flowers, Fennel seeds and Spinach leaves (suspensions of particles in fruit syrup).

Take 1 capful daily before a meal.

Available in bottles of 10 ml sample, 250 and 500 ml.

Internal use.

Tonic.

Visual.

Floradix® Formula
Herbal Iron Extract

Salus-Haus

Each 2 tsp. (10 ml) contains: Medicinal ingredients: Iron (ferrous) 7.5 mg, Vitamin B1 (Thiamine hydrochloride) 1.0 mg, Vitamin B2 (Riboflavin) 0.9 mg, Vitamin B6

(Pyridoxine hydrochloride) 0.5 mg, Folic acid 100 mcg, Vitamin B12 (Cyanocobalamin) 0.6 mcg in a base of extracts: Carrots, Nettles, Spinach, Quitch roots, Angelica roots, Fennel, Ocean kelp, African malva blossoms, Orange peel. Concentrates from: Pears, Red grapes, Black currants, Oranges, Blackberries, Cherries, Beetroots; Yeast extract (Saccharomyces cerevisiae), Honey, Rosehip extract and Wheat germ extract.

 Take 2 tsp. twice daily before meals. 1 measuring cap = 4 tsp.

Available in bottles of 10 ml trial size, 250, 500 and 700 ml.

Internal use. Organic. A natural-source food supplement with organic iron, yeast, herbs, fruit and honey.

Tonic.

Visual.

Floradix® Herbal Extract
Iron Tablets

Salus-Haus

Each tablet contains: Active ingredients: Yeast 120 mg, Niacinamide 10 mg, Vitamin C 10 mg, Iron 7 mg, Pyridoxine hydrochloride 2 mg, Riboflavin 1.5 mg, Thiamine 0.5 mg. Dry extracts of Spinach 32 mg, Rosehip 20 mg, Ocean kelp 16 mg, Fennel 12 mg, Angelica root 8 mg, Carrot 8 mg.

Take 1 tablet 3 times daily, before each meal.

Available in 84 tablets blister packed.

Internal use. Free of animal products.

Tablet.

Floradix® Liquid Calcium Magnesium-Zinc and Vitamin D

Salus-Haus

Each ml contains: Medicinal ingredients: Magnesium gluconate 69.03 mg, Magnesium citrate 33.93 mg, Calcium gluconate 35.10 mg, Calcium lactate 14.04 mg, Zinc citrate 0.39 mg, Vitamin D3 (Cholecalciferol) 6.66 IU. In a non-medicinal base containing herbal extracts of: Fennel, Camomile, Spinach plus natural tropical fruit concentrates.

Take 2 tbsp. daily or as directed by your physician.

Available in bottles of 10 ml trial size, 250 and 500 ml.

Internal use.

Tonic.

Visual.

Floradix® Multizyme
Herbal Tablets

Salus-Haus

Each tablet contains: Active ingredients: dry extracts of: Wormwood 30 mg, Anise 20 mg, Fennel 20 mg, Caraway 20 mg, Mint leaves 20 mg, Yarrow

20 mg, Aspergillus orycae-enzymes (equivalent to Pancreatin 4xNF XIII) 20 mg, Coriander 10 mg, Masterwort 10 mg, Bromelain 8 mg, 3.6 mg essential oil mixture from: Caraway oil 0.8 mg, Fennel oil 0.8 mg, Anise oil 0.8 mg, Peppermint oil 0.8 mg, Coriander oil 0.4 mg.

Take 2 tablets unchewed with liquid with each meal.

Available in 84 tablets per box.

Internal use. All ingredients are from natural sources and are selected in accordance with natural pharmaceutical principles.

Tablet.

FloraGuard® Echinacea Tincture

Flora Manufacturing & Distributing Ltd.

Contains: Certified organic Canadian-grown Echinacea angustifolia root (1 part) and Echinacea purpurea flower tops (3 parts) 1:7 (1 g Echinacea 7 ml tincture); made with top quality Canadian grain alcohol, 40% v/v. FloraGuard Echinacea tincture contains the extract of a total of 14 g of fresh Echinacea angustifolia root and fresh Echinacea purpurea flower tops per 100 ml of alcohol. The ratio of roots to flower tops is 1:3.

Take 15-30 drops with water every three hours until symptoms disappear, for up to 10 days.

Available in amber bottles of 50 and 100 ml.

Internal use. Organic.

Tincture.

If symptoms persist for more than 10 days, consult a qualified health practitioner. Not recommended for those with chronic immuno-deficiency illnesses. Pregnant or nursing mothers should consult a physician before taking any herbal medicine, as should parents intending to give it to their infants.

FloraLax® II
Natural Source Fibre with Oat Bran

Flora Manufacturing & Distributing Ltd.

Each tbsp. contains: Psyllium husks 2.3 g, Defatted flaxseed (certified organic) 2.5 g, Oat bran 0.2 g. Natural source fiber with oat bran.

Adults: take 1 tbsp. 1 to 3 times daily.
Children 6-12 years of age: give 1tbsp. 2 times daily.
Children under 6: consult your physician before administering.
Mix in at least 8 oz. of liquid with each dose. Mix well and drink immediately.

Available in amber bottle of 200 g.

Internal use. Bulk fiber.

Powder.

Do not swallow in dry form. Do not take within two hours of another medicine because the desired effect of the medi-

cine may be reduced. If allergic to psyllium seed husk, do not inhale or ingest this product. Do not use in the presence of abdominal pain, nausea, fever or vomiting (this refers to signs of appendicitis or inflamed bowel). If constipation persists for more than 7 days, consult your physician.

Visual.

FloraSil® (formerly "VegeSil")
Vegetal Silica Capsules

Flora Manufacturing & Distributing Ltd.

Each capsule contains: Atomized aqueous extract of: Spring horsetail (Equisetum arvense) 500 mg, supplying 9 to 11 mg of pure, soluble, organic Silica: in Vegicaps® (non- animal source, easily digested capsules).

Take 1-3 capsules daily with meals.

Available in amber bottles of 90, 180 and 360 capsules.

Internal use. Dr. Louis Kervran's patented Aqueous extract of Spring horsetail.

Vegetarin capsules.

Visual.

FloraSil® (formerly "VegeSil")
Vegetal Silica Powder

Flora Manufacturing & Distributing Ltd.

Contains: Atomized aqueous extract of: Spring horsetail

(Equisetum arvense) 50 g pure powder.

Take 1/4 to 1/2 tsp. once daily in 125 ml juice or warm water.

Available in 50 g.

Internal use. Dr. L. Kervran's patented atomized aqueous extract of Spring Horsetail.

Powder.

Formula F. L.W.®

Inno-Vite Inc.

Each tablet contains: Vitamins: Vitamin A (Palmitate) 4,000 IU, Vitamin E (d-alpha Tocopheryl succ.) 65 IU, Vitamin C (Ascorbic acid) 320 mg, Vitamin C (Calcium ascorbate) 80 mg, Vitamin B-1 (Thiamine hydrochloride) 20 mg, Vitamin B-2 (Riboflavin) 5 mg, Vitamin B-6 (Pyridoxine hydrochloride) 15 mg, Vitamin B-12 (Cobalamin) 25 mcg, Niacin 5 mg, Niacinamide 5 mg, Pantothenic acid (d-calcium pantothenate) 50 mg, Folic acid 0.04 mg, Biotin 10 mcg. Lipotropic factors: Choline (Bitartrate) 72.5 mg, Inositol 4 mg, dl-Methionine 24 mg. Minerals: Magnesium (oxide) 40 mg, Potassium (chloride) 20 mg, Potassium (citrate) 20 mg, Manganese (gluconate) 0.5 mg, Zinc (gluconate) 3 mg, Chromium (proteinate) 20 mcg, Selenium (proteinate) 25 mcg. Non-medicinal ingredients: Para-Aminobenzoic acid (P.A.B.A.) 25 mg, Betaine hydrochloride 12 mg, L-Cysteine hydrochloride 100 mg, Thymus concentrate 10 mg, Spleen concentrate 10 mg, Adrenal concentrate 10 mg.

Take 2 tablets daily with meals.

Available in 300 tablets.

Internal use.

Tablet.

Should not be taken within 2 hours of taking medicine.

Visual.

Frankincense
Essential Oil

Bach-Karooch Ltd.

Contains: Boswellia carteri 100%.

Two parts Essential oil must be diluted in 98 parts vegetable oil before applying to the skin. Consult Aromatherapy literature for specific methods of use and directions for each oil.

10 ml in amber bottle with child-resistant cap and one-drop insert.

Oil.

Caution: due to high concentration, all oils may be harmful if improperly used! External use only.

Fresh Cold Pressed Flaxseed Oil
High Lignan Content

Natural Factors® Nutritional Products Ltd.

Contains: Flaxseed oil with high lignan *content, d-alpha Tocopherol and gamma Tocopherol.

Flaxseed oil should be used within 6 weeks after opening the bottle.

Available in 270 ml.

Internal use. Contains no artificial preservatives, color, corn, dairy, gluten, starch, sweeteners or yeast. Natural Factors flaxseed oil, is pressed at low temperatures, without light or oxygen. This flaxseed oil is not refined, bleached, deodorized or filtered. Only organically grown seeds are used, without chemical fertilizers, pesticides or herbicides. Flaxseed oil is filled into black bottles to help keep it fresh, oxygen is then eliminated. *Lignans are natural phytochemicals found in high concentrations in Flaxseeds and this unique oil.

Oil.

Visual.

Fruit Chew Tangy Orange C 250 mg

Natural Factors® Nutritional Products Ltd.

Each tablet contains: Vitamin C 250 mg. Other ingredients: Bio sweet (fruit source™, naturally derived fruit sweeteners, maple crystals, natural flavor, natural color, Magnesium stearate, orange peel, citric acid, Rosehips, Rutin, Citrus bioflavonoids, Hesperidin, Silicon dioxide.

Take 1-6 tablets daily as directed by a physician.

Available in 90 and 180 chewable tablets.

Internal use. Contains no artificial preservatives, color, dairy starch, wheat or yeast.

Chewable tablets.

Visual.

Fruit Chew Tangy Orange C 500 mg

**Natural Factors®
Nutritional Products Ltd.**

Each tablet contains: Vitamin C 500 mg, in a natural base containing Bioflavonoids, Hesperidin, Rutin, Rosehips, Acerola and fruit flavors.

Take 1–3 tablets daily or as directed by a physician.

Available in 90 and 180 chewable tablets.

Internal use. Sweetened with Bio Sweet, a unique blend of sweeteners containing Fruit Source™, naturally derived fruit sweeteners and maple crystals. Four flavors include tangy orange, passion fruit, peach-mango, blueberry, raspberry, boysenberry and jungle juice. Contains no artificial preservatives, color, dairy, starch, wheat or yeast. Vegetarian formula.

Chewable tablet.

Visual.

Frutin®
Antacid Relief for Heartburn

New Nordic

Each tablet contains: Medicinal ingredients: Calcium carbonate (dolomite)

217 mg, Magnesium carbonate (dolomite) 183 mg. Non-medicinal ingredients: Pectin, Sorbitol, Peppermint flavoring.

Take 1 to 2 tablets as needed after meals, up to but no more than 8 tablets daily.

Available in amber bottle 60 tablets, dispenser: 30 tablets.

Internal use. Contains no aluminum or sodium bicarbonate. Sugar-free, no artificial colors or flavors. Safe for pregnant women.

Chewable tablet.

If you are taking another medicine, take the antacid tablets 2 hours before or 2 hours after taking your medicine. Should heartburn and/or acid indigestion persist after two consecutive weeks, or if symptoms recur, consult a physician for advice. Individuals with kidney disease should not take this product except on the advice of a doctor.

Visual.

Gallexier® Herbal Bitters

Salus-Haus

Each 100 ml contains: 82 g Herb extract (1:10) from Artichoke leaves 3.250 g, Dandelion herb 1.035 g, Gentian root 0.820 g, Turmeric root 0.590 g, Milfoil herb 0.590 g, Fennel 0.370 g, Camomile flowers 0.370 g, Blessed thistle herb 0.150 g, Buckbean leaves 0.075 g, Wormwood herb 0.035 g, Aromatic herbs 0.775 g, Fruit sugar 18 g. All ingredients of Gallexier are selected according to health food principles.

Take 1 measuring capful or 4 tsp. before meals as an appetizer or after meals as an aid to digestion.

Internal us. Contains no alcohol so it is suitable for those whose hepatic-bile system is particularly sensitive to alcohol.

Tonic.

Gamma Oil
Cold Pressed Evening Primrose Oil with Vitamin E

Quest Vitamins

Each capsule contains: Evening primrose oil 500 mg, Vitamin E (d-alpha Tocopherol) 14.9 IU. Contains 50 mg of Gamma linoleic acid (GLA) (10%) and 360 mg of Linoleic acid (LA). Capsule shell: Gelatin, Glycerin, Water.

Take 3 to 6 capsules daily with meals, or as directed by a health professional.

Available in 500 mg, 1000 mg and 1300 mg, 90 and 180 capsules.

Internal use. Solvent Free. Contains no artificial preservatives, colors, flavors or added sugar, starch, milk products, wheat or yeast.

Capsule.

Garlic Odorless

Nature's Herbs®

Each 556 mg capsule contains: Odorless garlic.

Take 3-4 capsules 3 times daily with a large glass of water.

Available in 100 capsules.

Internal use. Preservative-free.

Capsule.

Garlic-Black Walnut

Nature's Herbs®

Each 505 mg capsule contains: Odorless garlic, Black walnut, Fennel seed, and Cascara sagrada bark.

Take 2 capsules 3 times daily with a large glass of water for a period of 1 to 3 months.

Available in 100 capsules.

Internal use. Preservative-free.

Capsule.

Do not use if you have or develop diarrhea, loose stools, or abdominal pain. If you are pregnant, nursing, taking medication or have a medical conditions, consult your physician before using this product.

Garlic-Cayenne Herbal Formula

Nature's Herbs®

Each capsule contains: Odorless garlic and Cayenne.

Take 2-3 capsules 3 times daily with a large glass of water.

Available in 100 capsules.

Internal use. Preservative-free.

Capsule.

Gelsemium
Homeopathic Remedy

A. Nelson & Company Ltd.

Each pillule contains: Gelsemium sempervirens 6c.

Take 2 pillules every 2 hours for the first 6 doses, then 4 times daily for up to 5 days. Pillules should be sucked or chewed and taken between meals.

84 pillules/globules per bottle.

Internal use.

Pillule/globule.

Gentian
Bach Flower Remedy

Bach Flower Remedies® Ltd.

Contains: Gentiana amarella 5x in 27% grape alcohol solution.

Take 2 drops under the tongue 4 times daily or 2 drops in a small glass of spring water and sip at intervals.

10 ml with dropper.

Internal use.

Liquid.

Geranium Bourbon
Essential Oil

Bach-Karooch Ltd.

Contains: Pelargonium graveolens 100%.

Two parts Essential oil must be diluted in 98 parts vegetable oil before applying to the skin. Consult Aromatherapy literature for specific methods of use and directions for each oil.

10 ml in amber bottle with child-resistant cap and one-drop insert.

Oil.

Caution: due to high concentration, all oils may be harmful if improperly used! External use only.

Geriaforce®
A. Vogel
Ginkgo Biloba Tincture

Bioforce AG

Contains: Alcohol, Fresh wild Ginkgo biloba leaf.

Take 15-20 drops 3 times daily in a small amount of water, 15 minutes before meals. Salivate before swallowing.

Available in 50 ml.

Internal use.

Tincture.

Gincosan®

Pharmaton

Each capsule contains: Standardized Ginkgo biloba extract GK501™ 60 mg, adjusted to 24% ginkgo-flavone-glycosides and 6% terpene lactones (ginkgolides, bilobalide), Standardized Panax ginseng C.A. Meyer extract 100 mg. Non-medicinal: Mannitol, Silicon dioxide, Magnesium stearate. Capsule shell: Gelatin and natural color.

Take 2 capsules daily, 1 with breakfast and 1 with lunch.

Available in 30 and 60 capsules.

Contains no caffeine or artificial preservatives or colorants. Yeast free.

Capsule.

Not recommended for children under 12 years of age.

Ginger
Essential Oil

🏠 **Bach-Karooch Ltd.**

Contains: Zingiber officinale 100%.

Two parts Essential oil must be diluted in 98 parts vegetable oil before applying to the skin. Consult Aromatherapy literature for specific methods of use and directions for each oil.

10 ml in amber bottle with child-resistant cap and one-drop insert.

Oil.

Possible sensitization in some individuals.

Caution: due to high concentration, all oils may be harmful if improperly used! External use only.

Ginger Root

🏠 **Nature's Herbs®**

Each 535 mg capsule contains: Premium Ginger root.

Take 3 capsules 3 times daily with a large glass of water.

Available in 100 capsules.

Internal use. Preservative-free.

Capsule.

Ginger-Peppermint

🏠 **Nature's Herbs®**

Each capsule contains: Ginger root, Peppermint leaves, Cramp bark, Spearmint leaves, Wild yam root, Fennel seed, Catnip, Papaya leaves, Gelatin.

Take 2 capsules 3 times daily with a large glass of water.

Available in 100 capsules.

Internal use.

Capsule.

Ginkgo-Go!

🏠 **Wakunaga of America Co., Ltd.**

Each caplet contains: Ginkgo biloba extract 50:1 120 mg, standardized with ginkgo flavone glycosides 24%, terpene lactones 6%.

Take 1 caplet daily with a meal.

Available in 60 caplets.

Internal use.

Caplet.

Ginkgo Biloba
60 mg 24% Extract

🏠 **Natural Factors® Nutritional Products Ltd.**

Each tablet or capsule contains: Ginkgo leaf extract 60 mg, (24 % Ginkgo flavoglycosides) cellulose, Magnesium stearate.

Take 1 tablet or capsule daily or as directed by a physician.

Available in 30, 60 and 90 tablets or capsules.

Internal use. Contains no artificial preservatives, color, dairy, sweeteners, starch, wheat or yeast.

Capsule.

Tablet.

Visual.

Ginkgo Biloba

🏠 **Flora Manufacturing & Distributing Ltd.**

Each tablet contains: Standardized extract of: Ginkgo biloba (Ginkgo biloba) 1:50 40 mg standardized to contain 24% ginkgo flavon glycosides and 4% total terpenes lactones.

Take 1 or 2 tablets daily, before meals.

Available in amber bottles of 45 and 90 tablets.

Internal use. Contains no yeast, wheat, artificial colors or preservatives.

Tablet.

Visual.

Ginkgo Biloba

naka Sales Ltd.

Each capsule contains: Ginkgo biloba leaf extract 50:1 60 mg, Ginkgo biloba leaf extract, containing 24% Ginkgo flavone glycosides and 6% Ginkgo terpene lactones. Ginkgo biloba leaf 340 mg.

Take 1 capsule 3 times daily, or as directed by a professional.

Available in 120 capsules.

Internal use. Contains no artificial preservatives, colors, dairy, sweeteners, starch, wheat or yeast.

Capsule.

Ginkgo Biloba Extract

Nature's Herbs®

Contains: EuroQuality® extract of Ginkgo, standardized for .5% flavonoid glycosides, 6 g, in pure alpine spring water. Pure grain alcohol, 20% by volume.

Take 10-30 drops 3 times daily with water or juice. Shake well before using.

Available in 1 oz (30 ml).

Internal use.

Tincture.

Ginkgo Biloba Phyto GP-24

Albi Imports Ltd.

Each 400 mg capsule contains: Ginkgo biloba standardized extract (24% Ginkgo flavoglycosides, 6% terpenes) 60 mg, in a base of Ginkgo biloba leaf powder.

Take 1 capsule 3 times daily.

Available in 60, 120 and 360 capsules.

Internal use.

Capsule.

Visual.

Ginkgo Biloba Phytosome™

60 mg

Natural Factors® Nutritional Products Ltd.

Each capsule contains: Ginkgoselect™ Phytosome™ (Ginkgo leaf extract bound to phosphatidyl choline from

lecithin) 60 mg (24% Ginkgo flavoglycosides). Encapsulated in a gelatin capsule with vegetable grade Magnesium stearate (used as a lubricant).

Take 1 capsule daily or as directed by a physician.

Available in 60 and 90 capsules.

Internal use. Contains no artificial preservatives, color, dairy, sweeteners, starch, wheat or yeast.

Capsule.

Visual.

Ginkgo Power®

Nature's Herbs®

Each capsule contains: 40 mg Certified potency Ginkgo biloba extract (GBE) from Japan, concentrated and standardized for a minimum of preferred 24% flavonoid glycosides (of which 10% is quercetin and other naturally occurring flavonoids), in a synergistic base of holistic Ginkgo biloba leaf.

Take 3 capsules daily with meals.

Available in 50 capsules.

Internal use. Preservative-free. Three capsules are equivalent to about 6,000 mg or more of dry Ginkgo leaf.

Capsule.

Ginkoba®

Pharmaton

Each tablet contains: 40 mg of concentrated (50:1) extract from the leaves of the Ginkgo biloba tree. Non-medicinal: Lactose, Microcrystalline cellulose, Maize starch, Croscarmellose sodium, Magnesium stearate, Talc, Silicon dioxide, Film coating (Hydroxypropyl methylcellulose, Polyethylene glycol, Titanium oxide, Iron oxide, Sorbic acid, Polysorbate, Dimethyl polysiloxane).

Take 1 tablet 3 times daily at mealtimes.

Available in 54 tablets, blister packed.

Internal use.

Tablet.

Not recommended for children under 12 years of age. If you are taking a prescription medicine, are pregnant or lactating, contact a health professional before taking GINKOBA.

Ginsana® 100 and 200

Pharmaton

Each capsule contains: 100 mg or 200 mg of highly concentrated standardized Ginseng extract G115 (made from the roots of genuine Panax ginseng C. A. Meyer). Non-medicinal: canola oil, Lecithin, Vegetable stearin, Soybean oil, Beeswax, Soya lecithin, Ethylvanillin. Capsule shell: Gelatin, Glycerol, Ethylvanillin, natural color, Chlorophyll.

Ginsana® 100: take 2 capsules daily with breakfast or lunch. Ginsana® 200 take 1 capsule daily with breakfast or lunch.

Available in 30 and 60 capsules.

Internal use. Contains no caffeine, artificial preservatives or colorants. Yeast free.

Capsule.

Not recommended for children under 12 years of age.

Ginsana Liquid®

Pharmaton

Each 15 ml contains: 140 mg Standardized Ginseng extract G115 (made from roots of genuine Panax ginseng C.A. Meyer) with total ginsenoside concentration of 7.5 - 11%. Also contains Fructose, Sorbitol, Cherry and Tutti-fruiti flavors, Sodium citrate, Citric acid, Potassium sorbate, Sodium benzoate, Water.

Shake well before each use. Take 3 tsp. daily before or after a meal, best taken at breakfast.

250 ml.

Ginsana is produced using Ginseng Extract G115 which is standardized to guarantee a consistent potency and high level of quality. Contains no caffeine or artificial colorants.

Liquid.

Not recommended for children under 12 years of age.

Ginseng Enhanced Enrich I

naka Sales Ltd.

Each capsule contains: approximately 400 mg of: Siberian ginseng, Korean ginseng (extract), Ginkgo biloba (extract), Spirulina, Suma.

Take 1 or 2 capsules twice a day in between meals.

Available in 60 capsules.

Internal use.

Gelatin capsule.

Ginseng Herbal™

McZand® Herbal Inc.

Contains: Siberian ginseng (Eleutherococcus senticosus root) in a base of American ginseng root, Astragalus root, Ginkgo leaf, Cordonopsis root, Fo-Ti (Polygonum) root and Licorice root. Herbs extracted in distilled water, grain alcohol (ethyl alcohol USP) and vegetable glycerine. Contains 20-30% alcohol.

Take 2 capsules or 1 tsp. between meals 3-6 times daily.

Available in 117 ml and 472 ml liquid and 60 capsules.

Internal use.

Capsule.

Tincture.

Ginseng~Sarsaparilla

🏠 **Nature's Herbs®**

⚗️ Each 606 mg capsule contains: Siberian ginseng, Sarsaparilla, Norwegian kelp, Alfalfa, Periwinkle, Damiana, Licorice root, Black cohosh, Gelatin.

🤲 Take 3-4 capsules 3 times daily with a large glass of water.

📇 100 capsules.

🔲 Internal use. Preservative-free.

💊 Capsule.

⚠️ Do not consume Black cohosh (Cimicifuga racemosa) during pregnancy.

Ginseng~Saw Palmetto

🏠 **Nature's Herbs®**

⚗️ Each 454 mg capsule contains: Korean (Panax) ginseng, Saw palmetto berries, Damiana, Sarsaparilla and Cayenne.

🤲 Take 2 capsules 3 times daily, preferably at mealtimes.

📇 100 capsules.

🔲 Internal use. Preservative-free.

💊 Capsule.

Ginseng-Damiana Combination

🏠 **Nature's Herbs®**

⚗️ Each capsule contains: Siberian ginseng, Damiana

leaves, Sarsaparilla root, Bee pollen, Licorice root, Saw palmetto berries, Fo-Ti, Ginger root, Gelatin.

🤲 Take 2 capsules 3 times daily with a large glass of water.

📇 Available in 100 capsules.

🔲 Internal use.

💊 Capsule.

Glucosamine & Chondroitin Sulfate
500 mg

🏠 **Natural Factors® Nutritional Products Ltd.**

⚗️ Each capsule contains: Glucosamine sulfate 250 mg, Chondroitin sulfate 250 mg, in a gelatin capsule with vegetable grade Magnesium stearate (used as a lubricant) and rice protein.

🤲 Take 2-3 capsules daily or as directed by a physician.

📇 Available in 180 capsules.

🔲 Internal use. Contains no artificial preservatives, color, dairy, sweeteners, starch, wheat or yeast.

💊 Capsule.

📷 Visual.

Glucosamine Chondroitin Topical Gel

🏠 **Inno-Vite Inc.**

⚗️ Contains: Water, Carbomer, Acetyl glucosamine,

Chondroitin sulfate, Capsicum extract (Capsaicin), Chamomile extract, Devil's claw extract, Triethanolamine, Oil of Peppermint, Methyl paraben, Propyl paraben.

🤲 Apply to affected areas as required.

📇 Available in 120 ml.

🔲 External use.

🧴 Topical gel.

📷 Visual.

Glucosamine Sulfate

🏠 **naka Sales Ltd.**

⚗️ Each capsule contains: Glucosamine sulfate 500 mg, Magnesium stearate, Natural gelatin capsule shell.

🤲 Take 1 capsule 3 times daily, or as directed by a professional.

📇 Available in 120 capsules.

🔲 Internal use. Contains no artificial preservatives, colors, dairy, sweeteners, starch, wheat or yeast. Sodium free.

💊 Gelatin capsule.

Glucosamine Sulfate 1000 mg
Sodium Free

🏠 **Natural Factors® Nutritional Products Ltd.**

⚗️ Each capsule contains: Glucosamine sulfate 1000 mg.

Encapsulated in a gelatin capsule with vegetable grade Magnesium stearate (used as a lubricant). Sodium <0.050 mg, Potassium <100 mg.

Take 1-2 capsules daily or as directed by a physician.

Available in 60, 90 and 180 capsules.

Internal use. Contains no artificial preservatives, color, dairy, sweeteners, starch, wheat or yeast.

Capsule.

Visual.

Glucosamine Sulfate 500 mg

Sodium Free

**Natural Factors®
Nutritional Products Ltd.**

Each capsule contains: Glucosamine sulfate 500 mg in a gelatin capsule with vegetable grade Magnesium stearate (used as a lubricant) and rice protein. Sodium <0.025 mg, Potassium <50 mg.

Take 2-3 capsules daily or as directed by a physicians.

Available in 60, 90, 180 and 360 capsules.

Internal use. Contains no artificial preservatives, color, dairy, sweeteners, starch wheat or yeast.

Capsule.

Visual.

Golden Passage Menopause Formula®

Traditional Yin-Yang Herbals

Flora Manufacturing & Distributing Ltd.

Each 450 mg vegetarian capsule contains: Powdered aqueous extracts of: Ying yang huo (Epimedii, herba), Ba ji tian (Morindae officinalis, radix), Dang gui (Angelicae sinenses, radix), He shou wu (Polygoni multiflori, radix), Xian mao (Curculiginis orchioidis, rhizoma), Huang bai (Phellodendri, cortex), Zhi mu (Anemarrhenae asphodeloidis, rhizoma), Wu wei zi (Scisandrae chinensis, fructus), Gou qi zi (Lycii, fructus), Gan cao (Glycyrrhizae uralensis, radix); spray dried on a corn starch carrier. 1:5 aqueous extract.

Take 3-5 capsules daily with liquid. Take the capsules for 21 days. Stop for 7 days. Repeat cycle.

Available in 90 capsules of 450 mg each, in amber bottle.

Internal use. No preservatives added. To prevent contamination, do not drink directly from bottle. Shelf life after opening is 14 days. As presented by Dr. Malik Cotter (Diplomate of Oriental Medicine).

Vegetarian capsule.

Do not use when suffering from a cold, the flu or when digestion is disrupted. Pregnant women should exercise caution when taking this formula and not exceed the recommended amount.

Golden Passage Menopause Formula® Tonic

Traditional Yin-Yang Herbals

Flora Manufacturing & Distributing Ltd.

Each 500 ml contains: Purified water, aqueous extracts of: Ying yang huo (Epimedii, herba), Ba ji tian (Morindae officinalis, radix), Dang gui (Angelicae sinensis, radix), He shou wu (Polygoni multiflori, radix), Xian mao (Curculiginis orchioidis, rhizoma), Huang bai (Phellodendri, cortex), Zhi mu (Anemarrhenae asphodeloidis, rhizoma), Wu wei zi (Schisandrae chinensis, fructus), Gou qi zi (Lycii fructus), Gan cao (Glycyrrhizae uralensis, radix).

Shake the bottle well before use. Take 3 tbsp. two to three times daily. Dilute with warm water, if desired. Take the formula for 21 days. Stop for 7 days. Repeat cycle.

Available in 500 ml in amber bottle.

Internal use. No preservatives added. To prevent contamination, do not drink directly from bottle. Shelf life after opening is 14 days. As presented by Dr. Malik Cotter (Diplomate of Oriental Medicine).

Tonic.

Do not use when suffering from a cold, the flu or when digestion is disrupted. Pregnant women should exercise caution when taking this formula and should not exceed the recommended amount.

Golden Seal Root

🏠 **Nature's Herbs®**

⚗️ Each 540 mg capsule contains: Wild countryside® Goldenseal root.

🖐️ Take 1-2 capsules 3 times daily with a large glass of water.

📦 Available in 100 capsules.

Ⅱ Internal use. Preservative-free.

💊 Capsule.

Golden Seal Root Extract

🏠 **Nature's Herbs®**

⚗️ Contains: Extract of Wild countryside® Goldenseal root in filtered water and pure alcohol.

🖐️ Take 5-10 drops up to 3 times daily with water or juice. Shake well before using

📦 Available in 2 oz.

Ⅱ Internal use.

🖊️ Tincture.

Gorse

Bach Flower Remedy

🏠 **Bach Flower Remedies® Ltd.**

⚗️ Contains: Ulex europaeus 5x in 27% grape alcohol solution.

🖐️ Take 2 drops under the tongue 4 times daily or 2 drops in a small glass of spring water and sip at intervals.

📦 10 ml with dropper.

Ⅱ Internal use.

💧 Liquid.

Grape Seed Phytosome™

50 mg

🏠 **Natural Factors® Nutritional Products Ltd.**

⚗️ Each capsule contains: Leucoselect™ Phytosome™ (Grape seed extract bound to Phosphatidyl choline from lecithin) 50 mg (guaranteed minimum 95% leucoanthocyanins). Encapsulated in a gelatin capsule with vegetable grade Magnesium stearate (used as a lubricant).

🖐️ Take 1-2 capsules daily or as directed by a physician.

📦 Available in 60 capsules.

Ⅱ Internal use.

💊 Capsule.

📷 Visual.

Grape Seed Phytosome

🏠 **Nature's Herbs®**

⚗️ Each capsule contains: Grape seed phytosome 50 mg (concentrated and standardized at 95% polyphenols, including oligomeric proanthocyanidins).

🖐️ Take 2 capsules daily, preferably 1 with morning and evening meals.

📦 Available in 60 softgel capsules.

Ⅱ Internal use.

💊 Softgel capsule.

Grapefruit (White)

Essential Oil

🏠 **Bach-Karooch Ltd.**

⚗️ Contains: Citrus paradisi 100%.

🖐️ Two parts Essential oil must be diluted in 98 parts vegetable oil before applying to the skin. Consult Aromatherapy literature for specific methods of use and directions for each oil.

📦 10 ml in amber bottle with child-resistant cap and one-drop insert.

💧 Oil.

⚠️ Caution: due to high concentration, all oils may be harmful if improperly used! External use only.

Graphites

Homeopathic Remedy

🏠 **A. Nelson & Company Ltd.**

⚗️ Each pillule contains: Graphites 6c.

🖐️ Take 2 pillules every 2 hours for the first 6 doses, then 4 times daily for up to 5 days. Pillules should be sucked or chewed and taken between meals.

📦 84 pillules/globules per bottle.

Internal use.

Pillule/globule.

Green Kamut™ ®

Wheatgrass & Alfalfa Juice

Green Kamut Corporation

Each 330 mg vegetarian capsule contains: Certified organic (OCIA) combination of Kamut® Wheat grass juice and 35% mature Alfalfa leaf juice.

Powder: 2 tsp. 1-2 times daily, mixed with apple juice or water, shake or stir well. Capsules: 3 capsules daily. Take on empty stomach.

Available in 90 g/90 servings, 45 g/45 servings, 240 vegicaps/80 servings.

Grown in pure virgin soil high in the mountains of Utah, watered with mineral spring water. Grown seasonally. Three capsules is equivalent to 1 oz. of fresh juice. Dried below 88 °F. No binders, fillers or brown rice.

Capsule

Silky, light textured deep green powder that tastes like unsweetened tea.

Detoxification symptoms may occur.

Green Magma™ ®

Barley Grass Juice

Green Foods Corporation

Each tablet contains: Low temperature spray dried Barley grass juice, Maltodextrin, Brown rice.

Take 8 tablets or 1 tsp. of powder 1-3 times daily. Mix powder in 6-8 oz. of cold water or non-citrus/acid juice. Take on an empty stomach, first thing in morning and/or in between meals.

Available in powder or tablets. 5.3 oz. and 2.8 oz. 320 and 136 tablets.

This patented barley formulation utilizes a low heat, spray drying process which stabilizes enzyme activity and prevents oxidation of naturally occurring nutrients. Organically grown without any chemical fertilizers or pesticides.

Powder.

Tablet.

Green-Power™

Phytonutrient Blend with Beta-Carotene and Folic Acid

Nature's Herbs®

Each 531 mg capsule contains: Beta Carotene 25,000 IU, Folic Acid 400 mcg, *Green-Power Vegetable Blend 900 mg.
*Contains Carotene, Folic acid and chlorophyll rich vegetables: Certified potency Broccoli extract, Cabbage powder, Spinach powder, Parsley powder, Barley grass powder, Wheat grass powder, Alfalfa, Japanese Chlorella and Spirulina.

 Take 2-4 capsules daily.

60 capsules.

Internal use. Preservative-free.

Capsule.

Greens+™

Greens+™ Canada

Contains: Phosphatide complex (22% Phosphatidyl choline from 99% oil-free pure soy lecithin) 2120 mg, Organic Alfalfa, Barley & Wheat grass & whole Red beet juice powder 1543 mg, Hawaiian Spirulina pacific 1450 mg, Apple pectin fiber 1033 mg, Chlorella (cracked cell) 383 mg, organic Soy sprouts 383 mg, whole Brown rice powder 383 mg, 70 non-dairy probiotic cultures containing the lactobacilli (2.5 billion per serving): rhamnosus, acidophilus, bifidus, thermophilus, plantarum, bifido longum, and bifidobacterium bifidum in a base of FOS (fructo-oligosaccharides) 200 mg, Royal jelly (5% 10-HDA) 150 mg, Bee pollen 150 mg, Acerola berry juice powder 115 mg, organic Nova Scotia Pulse 33 mg.
*Standardized herbal extracts: Licorice root (15:1) 116 mg, Milk thistle (85.6% silymarin) 30:1 60 mg, Siberian E. ginseng (.5% eleutherosides) 12:1 60 mg, Ginkgo biloba (24% ginkgo flavonglycosides and 6% T. lactones) 50:1 20 mg, Japanese green tea (60% polyphenols) 2000:1 15 mg, European Bilberry (25% anthocyanidins) 100:1 10 mg, Grape seed extract (95% proanthocyanidins) 60:1 5 mg.
*Whole plant extract (in a special base of aromatic herbal glycosides).

Add 3 level tsp. of greens+ to one cup of pure water or juice. Take greens+ on an empty stomach or 15 minutes before breakfast. Begin with 1 tsp. daily and gradually increase to 3 tsp. daily.

255 g

Does not contain sugars, yeast, egg, coloring, alcohol, preservatives, salt, maltodextrin, gluten, corn, fats, oils, stabilizers, casein, or other milk derivatives. Non-irradiated. Each bottle is nitrogen flushed to preserve freshness.

Powder.

Visual.

GS Force™
Glucosamine Sulphate & Devil's Claw Extract

Prairie Naturals®

Each 500 mg capsule contains: Glucosamine sulfate 500 mg, Devil's claw (Harpogophytum procumbens) 20 mg, (secondary root extract, 5:1, equivalent to 100 mg of devil's claw root powder).

Take 1 capsule 3 times daily.

Available in 90, 180 and 360 capsules.

Internal use. Free of yeast, gluten, starch, soya, egg, dairy, artificial color, preservatives, solvents or alcohol.

Capsule.

Visual.

Hair-Force™

Prairie Naturals®

Each capsule contains: Vitamin C 133.3 mg, Vitamin A (Beta carotene) 3,333.3 IU, Vitamin D 370 IU, Pantothenic acid 166.7 mg, Vitamin B1 (Thiamine HCL) 10 mg, Vitamin B2 (Riboflavin) 10 mg, Vitamin B3 (Niacinamide) 15 mg, Vitamin B6 (Pyridoxine) 10 mg, Vitamin B12 (Cobalamine) 33.3 mcg, Folic acid 0.333 mg, Biotin 500 mcg. Lipotropic factors: Choline (bitartrate) 50 mg, Inositol 50 mg. Minerals: Zinc (citrate) 10 mg, Iodine (Potassium iodide) 0.33 mg, Selenium (amino acid chelate) 67 mcg. Amino acids: L-Cysteine 66.7 mg, L-Methionine 33.3 mg. Non-medicinal ingredients: PABA 66.7 mg.

Take 1-3 capsules daily or as directed by a physician.

Available in 90 and 180 capsule.

Internal use. Contains no yeast, gluten, starch, egg, dairy, artificial color or preservatives, solvents or alcohol.

Capsule.

Visual.

Hamamelis
Homeopathic Remedy

A. Nelson & Company Ltd.

Each pillule contains: Hamamelis virginiana 6c.

Take 2 pillules every 2 hours for the first 6 doses, then 4 times daily for up to 5 days. Pillules should be sucked or chewed and taken between meals.

84 pillules/globules per bottle.

Internal use.

Pillule/globule.

Harvestmoon™ Conditioner

Prairie Naturals®

Contains: Purified Water, Cetcaryl Alcohol, Hydrolyzed Grain Protein, Stearalkonium Chloride, Aloe Vera Extract, Glycerine, Pure Silica Extract 3%, Blended Combinations of Pure Natural Aromatic Oils: Sandwood, Geranium, Lavender, Rosemary, Purified Aqueous Extracts of Spring Horsetail (Silica), Oatstraw, Burdock, Chickweed, Black Walnut Leaves, White Willow, Lemon Grass, Nettles, Yarrow, Red Clover and Calendula, D-Panthenol, Allantonin from Comfrey, Grapefruit Seed Extract, Methyl Paraben, Fragrance of Natural Aromatic Oils.

Apply to wet hair. Massage gently into the hair and scalp and let penetrate for several minutes. Rinse with lukewarm water.

Available in 250 ml bottles.

External use only. Enviro-wise and biodegradable. Not tested on animals.

Shampoo.

Harvestmoon™ Shampoo

⌂ **Prairie Naturals®**

⚗ Contains: Purified water, Disodium oleamido sulfosucinates, Cocoamide DEA/Cocamido propyl betaine, Maize gluten amino acids, D-panthenol, PEG-7 glyceryl cocoate, Pure silica extract 3%, Ascorbic acid, Allantoin, Vitamin E, Jojoba oil, Papaya extract, Aloe vera extract, Aromatic oils: Sandalwood, Geranium Lavender, Rosemary, Purified aqueous extracts of: Spring horsetail (Silica), Oatstraw, Burdock, Chickweed, Black walnut leaves, White willow, Lemon grass, Nettles, Yarrow, Red clover and Calendula, D-Panthenol, Allantoin from comfrey, Grapefruit seed extract, Methyl paraben, fragrance of natural aromatic oils.

✍ Apply to wet hair. Massage gently into the hair and scalp and let penetrate for several minutes. Rinse with lukewarm water. Follow with a suitable Prairie Naturals Conditioner and styling aid.

▣ Available in 125 and 500 ml bottles.

Ⓘ External use only. Enviro-wise and biodegradable. Not tested on animals.

◊ Shampoo.

Hawaiian Energizer

⌂ **Nutrex® Inc.**

⚗ Each 500 mg tablet contains: Certified organic Spirulina, Siberian ginseng, Bee pollen. Drink mix contains: Soy protein isolate, Banana, Complex carbohydrate from Tapioca yam, Fruitsource® fruit and whole grain sweetener, Certified organic Hawaiian Spirulina pacifica™, Apple fiber, Organic green Papaya, Hawaiian taro, Bee pollen, Ginseng, Ginger and the following Vitamins and Minerals: Vitamin C (ascorbic acid and acerola), Calcium carbonate, Magnesium oxide, Dicalcium phosphate, d alpha-Tocopherol acetate (natural Vitamin E), Copper gluconate, Biotin, Niacinamide (B3), Zinc oxide, Calcium pantothenate, Phytonadione (Vitamin K), Ergocalciferol (Vitamin D), Pyridoxine HCL (B6), Riboflavin, Thiamine HCl (B1), Cyanocobalamin (B12), Folic acid, Potassium iodide.

✍ Take 6 or more tablets or 2 tbsp. daily. Drink mix: blend with juice, soy milk or other beverage.

▣ Available in 90 tablets or 16 oz. drink mix.

Ⓘ Internal use.

⊸ Powder.

⊘ Tablet.

Hawthorn Juice

⌂ **W. Schoenenberger**

⚗ Contains: Pure natural pressed herb and plant juice from organically grown Hawthorn.

✍ Shake bottle before use. Take 3 or 4 times daily before meals 1 tbsp. diluted in water, milk or tea, one part juice to six parts liquid. For children 1 tsp. instead of tbsp. Unopened bottle will keep indefinitely: opened, for 6 days.

▣ Amber bottle of 5.5 fl. oz.

Ⓘ Internal use. Organically grown in nearly ideal conditions in the Black Forest & Swabian uplands, where the air is pure. The plants are gathered at the moment when their production of valuable ingredients is at its peak. The juices are extracted by specially designed hydraulic presses that ensure maximum recovery of all essential elements, making certain that not more than 2-3 hours elapse between harvesting, pressing and bottling.

◊ Cellular plant juice.

Hawthorn Phytosome

⌂ **Nature's Herbs®**

⚗ Each capsule contains: Hawthorn phytosome 100 mg (concentrated and standardized at 8% isovitexin).

✍ Take 2 capsules daily, preferably 1 with morning and evening meals.

▣ Available in 60 softgel capsules.

Ⓘ Internal use.

▭ Softgel capsule.

HB-CRC 11
Garlic Plus

⌂ naka Sales Ltd.

Each capsule contains approximately 515 mg of: Garlic, Guggul, Parsley, Fennel, Hawthorn, Ginger, Capsicum.

Take 1 or 2 capsules with each meal.

Available in 150 capsules.

Internal use. Odorless and non bloating.

Capsule.

Healthy Trinity
Probiotic Microflora

Natren™ Inc.

Each capsule contains: a minimum of one billion Lactobacillus acidophilus NAS Super strain, one billion Bifidobacterium bifidum Malyoth Super strain, and one billion Lactobacillus bulgaricus LB-51 Super strain.

Take 1 capsule daily with a meal.

Available in 30 and 90 capsules.

Internal use.

Capsule.

Some detoxification may occur.

Heather
Bach Flower Remedy

Bach Flower Remedies® Ltd.

Contains: Calluna vulgaris 5x in 27% grape alcohol solution.

Take 2 drops under the tongue 4 times daily or 2 drops in a small glass of spring water and sip at intervals.

10 ml with dropper.

Internal use.

Liquid.

Heaven Grade Korean Red Ginseng

Albi Imports Ltd.

Each tablet contains: Korean red ginseng extract powder (standardized extract, Rg=27 1%) 100 mg, total Ginsenosides, Korean red ginseng root powder 400 mg.

Take 1–3 tablets daily, preferably before morning meal.

50 tablets. Available in capsules, cream, teas, powder, liquid extract in various strengths and forms.

Internal use. Made from the six year old roots.

Liquid extract.

Tablet.

Visual.

Hemorrhoid Cream
Homeopathic Cream

A. Nelson & Company Ltd.

Contains: Extracts of organically grown Aesculus hippocastanum 1x 2.4%,

Calendula officinalis 1x 2.4%, Hamamelis virginica 1x 2.4% and Paeonia officinalis 1x 2.4% in a base of almond oil, avocado oil and cocoa butter.

Clean affected area, then apply cream to area thoroughly.

27 g tube.

External use. Organic. Not tested on animals.

Cream.

Avoid contact with eyes. If symptoms persist, consult a physician.

Hepar Sulph.
Homeopathic Remedy

A. Nelson & Company Ltd.

Each pillule contains: Hepar sulphuris calcareum 6c.

Take 2 pillules every 2 hours for the first 6 doses, then 4 times daily for up to 5 days. Pillules should be sucked or chewed and taken between meals.

84 pillules/globules per bottle.

Internal use.

Pillule/globule.

Herbal Calm®

Nature's Herbs®

Each capsule contains: Valerian root extract 4:1, Passion flower extract 4:1, Scullcap extract 4:1, Hops and Kava Kava.

Take 3-4 capsules at bedtime with a large glass of water.

Available in 100 capsules.

Internal use. Preservative-free.

Capsule.

Do not use when driving a motor vehicle or operating machinery. Do not use if you are taking sedatives or tranquilizers without first consulting a health care professional.

Herbal Eyebright

Nature's Herbs®

Each 434 mg capsule contains: Eyebright, Goldenseal root, Bayberry bark, Red raspberry leaves and Cayenne.

Take 3 capsules 3 times daily with a large glass of water.

Available in 100 capsules.

Internal use. Preservatives-free.

Capsule.

Herbal Fibre

Albi Imports Ltd.

Each capsule contains: Psyllium husks, Chinese licorice root, Butternut bark, Black walnut, Chinese rhubarb, Bentonite, Fennel seed.

Take 1–2 capsules before morning meal or as required,

or add 1 tsp. to a full glass of water upon waking. Mix thoroughly and follow with another full glass of water.

Available in 90, 180 and 500 capsules, and 250 g and 454 g powder.

Internal use.

Capsule.

Powder.

May experience a sense of fullness after taking.

Herbal Juice Therapy Kit: 20-day Liver Cleanse

Schoenenberger Juices

Flora Manufacturing & Distributing Ltd.

Each kit contains: Black radish juice, Dandelion juice, Peppermint tea and Fig syrup.

Follow instructions in kit.

Each kit includes: 1 bottle of Fig syrup, 3 bottles of Black radish juice, 2 bottles of Dandelion juice, 40 Peppermint tea bags. Each bottle of juice contains 160 ml of plant juice.

Internal use. Each kit contains: 1 bottle Fig syrup, 40 Peppermint tea bags, 3 bottles black Radish juice and 2 bottles Dandelion juice. Keep opened bottles refrigerated.

Herbal Tea.

Plant juices.

Tonic.

Herbal Juice Therapy Kit: 24-day Nerval Tonic Program

Schoenenberger Juices

Flora Manufacturing & Distributing Ltd.

Each kit contains: Nerval tonic tea, St. John's wort juice, Valerian juice.

Follow instructions in kit.

Each kit includes: 4 bottles of St. John's wort juice, 2 bottles of Valerian juice and 48 Nerval Tonic tea bags. Each bottle of juice contains 160 ml of plant juice.

Internal use.

Herbal Tea.

Plant juice.

Tonic.

Herbal Laxative Formula

Quest Vitamins

Each caplet contains: Cascara sagrada bark (provided by 50 mg P.E. 1:7) 350 mg, Rhubarb root (Rheum officinale L) (provided by 30 mg P.E. 1:4) 120 mg, in a specially prepared non-medicinal herbal base containing Cayenne, Ginger root, Licorice root and Marshmallow root; Calcium phosphate, Croscarmellose sodium, Microcrystalline cellulose, Magnesium stearate (vegetable source), Vegetable stearin. Cell coat: Vegetable cellulose complex.

Take 2 caplets daily as needed, or as directed by a health professional.

Available in 60 caplets.

Internal use.

Caplet.

Do not use this product in the presence of abdominal pain, nausea, fever or vomiting or within two hours of another medicine since the desired effect of the other medicine may be reduced. Extended use of any laxative can cause dependence for bowel function, do not take for more than one week unless directed by a health professional.

Herbal Migraine Formula

Quest Vitamins

Each caplet contains: Feverfew leaf powder (contains not less than 0.2% parthenolides) 125 mg in a specially prepared non-medicinal herbal base of Blue vervain, Kelp, Milk thistle, Peppermint leaf, Red raspberry leaf, Skullcap and Wood betony; Calcium phosphate, Croscarmellose sodium, Microcrystalline cellulose, Vegetable stearin, Magnesium stearate (vegetable source). CellCote Coating: Vegetable cellulose complex.

Take 1 or 2 caplets daily or as directed by a health professional.

Available in 60 caplets.

Internal use.

Caplet.

Do not use this product during pregnancy or lactation, or if sore or ulcerated mouth occurs. Do not use for more than four months except on the advice of a health professional.

Herbal Relaxant Formula

Quest Vitamins

Each caplet contains: Valerian root (provided by 100 mg P.E. 1:5 standardized to contain 0.8% valerenic acid) 500 mg, Chamomile flower (Chamomilla recutita L) (provided by 50 mg P.E. 1:4 standardized to contain 1% apigenin) 200 mg. Non-medicinal herbal base: Ginger root, Hops, Marshmallow root, and Scullcap; Calcium phosphate, Croscarmellose sodium, Magnesium stearate (vegetable source), Microcrystalline cellulose, Vegetable stearin.

Take 2 caplets at bedtime, or as directed by a health professional.

Available in 60 caplets.

Internal use.

Caplet.

Avoid alcoholic beverages and using machinery, driving or activities requiring alertness while using this product. Do not exceed the recommended dose or take this product while pregnant or breast feeding, unless directed by a health professional. If sleeplessness persists continuously for more than 2 weeks, consult your health professional. Insomnia may be a symptom of serious underlying medical illness.

Herbal Women's Formula

Quest Vitamins

Each caplet contains: White willow bark powder (provided by 85 mg P.E. 1:12 standardized to contain 11% salicin) 1000 mg, Valerian root (provided by 40 mg P.E. 1:5 standardized to contain 0.8% valerenic acid) 200 mg, Chamomile flower (Chamomilla recutita L) (provided by 20 mg P.E. 1:4 standardized to contain 1% apigenin) 80 mg, Uva ursi leaf (provided by 50 mg P.E. 1:4 standardized to contain 10% arbutin) 200 mg, Juniper berry (provided by 80 mg P.E. 1:4) 320 mg, Parsley root (provided by 40 mg P.E. 1:4) 160 mg in a specially prepared non-medicinal herbal base containing Bladderwack, Garlic, Kelp, Licorice root, Passion flower, Raspberry leaf, Saw palmetto berry, Squaw vine, Wild yam root; Calcium phosphate, Croscarmellose sodium, Magnesium stearate (vegetable source), Microcrystalline cellulose, Silicon dioxide.

Take 2 caplets 3 times daily with meals, or as directed by a health professional.

Available in 30 caplets.

Internal use.

Caplet.

For occasional use only. It is hazardous to exceed the maximum recommended dose unless advised by a physician. May cause drowsiness: do not drive or engage in activities requiring alertness. Do not use during pregnancy and avoid alcoholic beverages. Consult a physician if the underlying condition requires continued use for more than five days.

Herbon™ Adventurous Tingle™Herbal Cough Drops

🏠 **Herbon Naturals, Inc.**

⚗️ Each cough drop contains in 1:1 liquid extracts: organic Echinacea 250 mg, Licorice root 3 mg, Menthol 5 mg, Bee propolis 2 mg, Sucrose, Corn syrup, Citric acid and Natural orange flavoring.

👐 Suck 6-7 drops daily.

📦 Available in 18 drops per package.

ℹ️ Herbon drops are available in three more unique formulations Wild cherry, Glacial mint and Lemon honey. Each of these contain 100 mg of organic Echinacea in combination with other medicinal herbs.

⊘ Lozenge.

⚠️ If dry cough worsens, persists for more than 7 days, or is accompanied by a high fever, consult a physician.

📷 Visual.

Hi Potency B Complex
50 mg

🏠 **Natural Factors® Nutritional Products Ltd.**

⚗️ Each capsule contains: Vitamin B-1 (Thiamine hydrochloride) 50 mg, Vitamin B-2 (Riboflavin) 50 mg, Niacinamide 50 mg, Vitamin B-6 (Pyridoxine hydrochloride) 50 mg, Vitamin B-12 (Cyanocobalamin) 50 mcg, Biotin 60 mcg, Folic acid 1 mg, d-Pantothenic acid 50 mg. Lipotropic factors: Choline bitartrate 50 mg, Inositol 50 mg. Non-medicinal ingredient: Para Amino Benzoic acid 50 mg.

👐 Take 1 capsule daily or as directed by a physician.

📦 Available in 60, 90 and 180 capsules.

ℹ️ Internal use. Contains no artificial preservatives, color, corn, dairy, gluten, soya, starch, sweeteners or yeast.

💊 Capsule.

📷 Visual.

Hi Potency B Compound
50 mg

🏠 **Natural Factors® Nutritional Products Ltd.**

⚗️ Each tablet contains: Vitamin B-1 (Thiamine hydrochloride) 50 mg, Vitamin B-2 (Riboflavin) 50 mg, Niacinamide 50 mg, Vitamin B-6 (Pyridoxine hydrochloride) 50 mg, Vitamin B-12 (Cyanocobalamin) 50 mcg, Biotin 50 mcg, Folic acid 1 mg, d-Pantothenic acid 50 mg. Lipotropic factors: Choline bitartrate 50 mg, Inositol 50 mg. Non-medicinal ingredient: Para Amino Benzoic acid 50 mg.

👐 Take 1 tablet daily or as directed by a physician.

📦 Available in 60, 90 and 180 tablets.

ℹ️ Internal use. Contains no artificial preservatives, color, corn, dairy, gluten, soya, starch, sweeteners or yeast.

⊘ Tablet.

📷 Visual.

Hi Potency Multi
Vegetarian Formula

🏠 **Natural Factors® Nutritional Products Ltd.**

⚗️ Each tablet contains: Beta carotene (Provitamin A) 10,000 IU, Vitamin D 3 (Lanolin) 400 IU, Vitamin B-1 (Thiamine hydrochloride) 50 mg, Vitamin B-2 (Riboflavin) 50 mg, Niacinamide 50 mg, Vitamin B-6 (Pyridoxine hydrochloride) 50 mg, Vitamin B-12 (Cyanocobalamin) 50 mcg, Pantothenic acid (Calcium pantothenate) 50 mg, Folic acid 1.0 mg, Biotin 50 mcg, Vitamin C (Ascorbic acid) 200 mg, Vitamin E (d-alpha Tocopheryl succinate) 100 IU. Lipotropic factors: Choline bitartrate 50 mg, Inositol 50 mg, Methionine 50 mg. Minerals: Calcium (HVP* chelate) 125 mg, Magnesium (HVP* chelate) 50 mg, Iron (HVP* chelate) 10 mg, Potassium (citrate) 10 mg, Zinc (citrate) 10 mg, Manganese (citrate) 1 mg, Iodine (potassium/kelp) 0.1 mg, Chromium (HVP* chelate) 25 mcg, Molybdenum (HVP* chelate) 25 mcg, Selenium (HVP* chelate) 25 mcg. Non-medicinal ingredients: Para Amino Benzoic acid 50 mg, Citrus bioflavonoids 50 mg, Hesperidin 10 mg, Betaine hydrochloride 50 mg, Papain 10 mg, *Hydrolyzed vegetable (rice) protein.

Take 1 tablet daily or as directed by a physician.

Available in 60, 90 and 180 tablets.

Internal use. Contains no artificial preservatives color, dairy, sweeteners, starch, wheat or yeast.

Tablet.

There is enough iron in this product to seriously harm a child.

Visual.

HMB™ (U.S.)

EAS

Each capsule contains: Calcium beta-hydroxy Beta-methylbutyrate monohydrate (HMB) 250 mg, Gelatin, Monopotassium phosphate, Water.

Take 4 capsules 3 times daily with meals.

Available in 120 and 360 capsules.

Internal use. HMB is an amino acid metabolite derived from the branched-chain amino acid leucine.

Capsule.

Visual.

Holistic Horizon's Starter Kit®

Holistic Horizons

Starter kit contains: 2 Intestinal bulking agent II (340 g), 1 Herbal enhancement formula (100 tablets), 1 DDS Acidophilus (100 capsules).

Follow instructions on kit.

Products are sold separately or in a starter kit.

Internal use.

Capsule.

Powder.

Tablet.

Some women experience a change of menstrual cycle.

Do not use products during pregnancy or if any of the following conditions exist; Inflammatory bowel disease, Crohn's disease, Regional ileitis or Ulcerative colitis. Do not use the program if taking Salicylates, or on prescription medication. Do not take if you are on drugs containing Digitalis or Nitrofuration, as the Psyllium present in either bulking agent may combine with these drugs.

Visual.

Holly
Bach Flower Remedy

Bach Flower Remedies® Ltd.

Contains: Ilex aquifolium 5x in 27% grape alcohol solution.

Take 2 drops under the tongue 4 times daily or 2 drops in a small glass of spring water and sip at intervals.

10 ml with dropper.

Internal use

Liquid.

Honeysuckle
Bach Flower Remedy

Bach Flower Remedies® Ltd.

Contains: Lonicera caprifolium 5x in 27% grape alcohol solution.

Take 2 drops under the tongue 4 times daily or 2 drops in a small glass of spring water and sip at intervals.

10 ml with dropper.

Internal use.

Liquid.

Hops-Valerian Herbal Formula

Nature's Herbs®

Each 404 mg capsule contains: Hops, Valerian root and Scullcap.

Take 3-4 capsules 3 times daily or 4-6 capsules upon retiring with a large glass of water.

Available in 100 capsules.

Internal use. Preservative-free.

Capsule.

Do not use when driving a motor vehicle or operating machinery. Do not use if you are taking sedatives or tranquilizers without first consulting a health care professional.

Hornbeam

Bach Flower Remedy

Bach Flower Remedies® Ltd.

Contains: Carpinus betulus 5x in 27% grape alcohol solution.

Take 2 drops under the tongue 4 times daily or 2 drops in a small glass of spring water and sip at intervals.

10 ml with dropper.

Internal use.

Liquid.

Horse Chestnut Power™

Nature's Herbs®

Each capsule contains: 257 mg certified potency Horse chestnut extract concentrated and standardized for a minimum of 18-22% triterpenoid glycosides (calculated as escin), synergistically combined with Butcher's broom, Ginger root and Rutin.

Take 1 capsule both with morning and evening meals.

Available in 60 capsules.

Internal use. Preservative-free.

Capsule.

Horsetail Tincture

Salus-Haus

Each 10 g tincture contains: 10 g extract derived from 2 g Horsetail plant.

Unless otherwise directed, take 10-20 drops diluted in a small amount of liquid 2-3 times daily.

Available in 50 ml, includes a dropper.

Internal use. Salus herbal tinctures are made in accordance with strictest health food principles, using natural ingredients only.

Tincture.

HSC Herbal Decongestant-Expectorant

Vita Health Co. Ltd.

Each capsule contains: Ma huang (Ephedra sinica) 50 mg, Wild horehound leaf (Marrubium vulgarae) 150 mg, Thyme herb (Thymus vulgaris) 400 mg, Coltsfoot leaf (Tussilago farfara) 50 mg, Mullein leaf (Verbascum thapsus) 50 mg, Cayenne (Capsicum minimum) 1.125 mg, Marshmallow root (Althaea officinalis) 9 mg, Slippery elm bark (Ulmus fulva) 9 mg.

Take 2 capsules every 6 hours (maximum 8 daily).

Available in 90 capsules.

Internal use.

Capsule.

Ephedra: large doses may lead to insomnia, dry mouth, nervousness, headache, dizziness, palpitations, skin flushing, tingling and vomiting.

Not recommended during pregnancy and lactation, or in cases of heart disease, thyroid disease, high blood pressure, diabetes, glaucoma, difficulty in urination due to prostate enlargement, recent or concurrent use of MAO inhibitors. It is also not recommended for those who have cardiac insufficiency or enterocolitis., or for children under 18.

HSC Herbal Insomnia Formula

Vita Health Co. Ltd.

Each tablet contains: Valerian extract (Valerian officinalis) 50 mg, Passion flower herb (Passiflora incarnata) 80 mg, Chamomile flower (Maticaria recutita) 60 mg, Hops flower (Humulus lupulus) 50 mg, Mistletoe herb (Viscum album) 50 mg, Wild lettuce leaf (Lactuca virosa) 40 mg.

Take 1-2 tablets in the evening.

Available in 100 tablets.

Internal use. Vegetarian.

Tablet.

Not recommended during pregnancy and lactation, or in cases of depression.

HSC Nomigraine™

🏠 **Vita Health Co. Ltd.**

⚗️ Each caplet contains: 125 mg of Feverfew extract standardized to a minimum of 0.2% parthenolide.

🖐️ Take 1-2 caplets daily with water.

📦 Available in 60 caplets.

🔲 Vegetarian. Internal use.

💊 Caplet.

⚠️ Discontinue use if sore or ulcerated mouth occurs.

✋ Not recommended during pregnancy and lactation, or in cases of hypersensitivity to plants in the daisy family.

HSC St. John's Wort

🏠 **Vita Health Co. Ltd.**

⚗️ Each caplet contains: St. John's wort (Hypericum perforatum) standardized extracts 1:5 with 0.3% hypericins 300 mg (equivalent to 1500 mg St. John's wort).

🖐️ Take 3 caplets daily.

📦 Available in 60 caplets per bottle.

🔲 Internal use. Suitable for vegetarians.

💊 Caplet.

⚠️ Photosensitization may occur, may cause drowsiness. Do not drive or engage in activities requiring alertness.

✋ Avoid alcoholic beverages. Consult with physician if currently taking Monoamine oxidase (MAO) inhibitor drugs. Safety during pregnancy and lactation has not been determined.

HSC Stomach-Ease® Herbal Laxative

🏠 **Vita Health Co. Ltd.**

⚗️ Each tablet contains: Senna leaves (Cassia angustifolia) 240 mg, Cascara sagrada bark (Rhamnus purshiana) 150 mg, Licorice root (Glycyrrhiza glabra) 30 mg, Juniper berries (Juniperus communis) 8 mg, Rhubarb root (Rheum palmatum) 8 mg, Gentian root (Gentiana lutea) 8 mg, Buchu leaves (Barosma betulina) 4 mg, Oil of Peppermint 0.2 mg.

🖐️ Take 1 tablet at bedtime, or as required.

📦 Available in 100 tablets and 250 tablets.

🔲 Internal use. Suitable for vegetarians.

💊 Tablet.

⚠️ Long term use may cause potassium deficiency. Frequent and continuous use may lead to dependency and development of an atonic non-functioning colon.

✋ Not recommended during pregnancy and lactation, or in cases of undiagnosed abdominal symptoms, inflammatory bowel disease, appendicitis, hypokalemia, intestinal hemorrhage, gastric or duodenal ulcers, hypertension, liver cirrhosis or kidney problems. Do not take a laxative within 2 hours of other medication because the desired effect of the other medication may be reduced.

Hyland's™ Gas Remedy

🏠 **Standard Homeopathic and P&S Laboratories**

⚗️ Contains: Nux moschata 3x, Asafoetida 3x, Ignatia 3x, Lycopodium 6x.

🖐️ Dissolve 2-3 tablets under tongue every 4 hours or as needed. Children's dosage is 1/2 the adult dosage.

📦 Available in bottles of 100 tablets.

🔲 Internal use. Safe for adults & children and can be used in conjunction with other medications.

⊘ Sub-lingual lactose tablet.

Hyland's™ Indigestion

🏠 **Standard Homeopathic and P&S Laboratories**

⚗️ Contains: Cinchona off. 3x, Hydrastis can. 3x, Phosphoricum acidum 3x, Kali bichromicum 3x.

🖐️ Dissolve 2-3 tablets under tongue every 4 hours or as needed. Children's dosage is 1/2 the adult dosage.

Available in bottles of 100 tablets.

Internal use. Safe for adults & children and can be used in conjunction with other medications.

Sublingual lactose tablet.

Hyland's™ Motion Sickness

Standard Homeopathic and P&S Laboratories

Contains: Nux vomica 6x, Tabacum 6x, Petroleum 12x, Cocculus indicus 30x.

Dissolve 2-3 tablets under tongue every 4 hours or as needed. Children's dosage is 1/2 the adult dosage.

Available in bottles of 50 tablets.

Internal use. Safe for adults & children and can be used in conjunction with other medications.

Sublingual lactose tablet.

Hyland's™ Upset Stomach

Standard Homeopathic and P&S Laboratories

Contains: Nux vomica 3x, Carbo vegetabilis 3x.

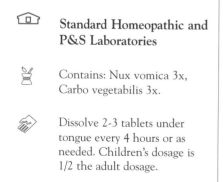

Dissolve 2-3 tablets under tongue every 4 hours or as needed. Children's dosage is 1/2 the adult dosage.

Available in bottles of 100 tablets.

Internal use. Safe for adults & children and can be used in conjunction with other medications.

Sublingual lactose tablet.

Hypercal®
Hypericum/Calendula Homeopathic Cream

A. Nelson & Company Ltd.

Contains: Extracts of organically grown Hypericum perforatum 1x 4.5% and Calendula officinalis 1x 4.5% in a base of almond oil, avocado oil and cocoa butter.

Clean affected area, then apply cream to area thoroughly. Cover with bandage if necessary.

27 g tube.

External use. Organic. Not tested on animals.

Cream.

Avoid contact with eyes. If symptoms persist, consult a physician.

Hypericum
Homeopathic Remedy

A. Nelson & Company Ltd.

Each pillule contains: Hypericum perforatum 6c.

Take 2 pillules every 2 hours

for the first 6 doses, then 4 times daily for up to 5 days. Pillules should be sucked or chewed and taken between meals.

84 pillules/globules per bottle.

Internal use.

Pillule/globule.

Hyssop
Essential Oil

Bach-Karooch Ltd.

Contains: Hyssopus officinalis 100%.

Two parts Essential oil must be diluted in 98 parts vegetable oil before applying to the skin. Consult Aromatherapy literature for specific methods of use and directions for each oil.

10 ml in amber bottle with child-resistant cap and one-drop insert.

Oil.

Caution: due to high concentration, all oils may be harmful if improperly used!
External use only. Avoid during pregnancy or if epileptic. Do not use if you have high blood pressure.

Ignatia
Homeopathic Remedy

A. Nelson & Company Ltd.

Each pillule contains: Ignatia amara 6c.

Take 2 pillules every 2 hours for the first 6 doses, then 4 times daily for up to 5 days. Pillules should be sucked or chewed and taken between meals.

84 pillules/globules per bottle.

Internal use.

Pillule/globule.

IMMU-Cholesterol
Black Seed, Garlic & Lecithin

Kare & Hope Inc.

Each capsule contains: Black seed 250 mg, Garlic (Pur-Gar) 275 mg, Lecithin (PhosphatidylCholine) 360 mg.

Take 3 capsules twice daily or as recommended by a health care professional.

100 capsules.

No added sugar, salt, preservatives or any artificial chemicals.

Capsule.

Impatiens
Bach Flower Remedy

Bach Flower Remedies® Ltd.

Contains: Impatiens glandulifera 5x in 27% grape alcohol solution.

Take 2 drops under the tongue 4 times daily or 2 drops in a small glass of spring water and sip at intervals.

10 ml with dropper.

Internal use.

Liquid.

Inca-Rice™ Golden Quinoa

Artesian Acres Inc.

Contains: Golden Quinoa.

Food. Inca-Rice™ Golden Quinoa is organically grown in Canada, lightly pearled to preserve its live properties (it will germinate). Wheat and gluten-free.

Visual.

Inflam-Aid®

Nature's Herbs®

Each 6 capsules contains: Vitamin C 1000 mg, natural Vitamin E (d-alpha Tocopherol succinate) 400 IU, standardized Ginger root (6-8% oils) and Ginger root 1000 mg, Certified potency White willow bark root (standardized for 15% salicin) 400 mg, Certified potency Turmeric herb (standardized for 95% Curcumin) 600 mg, Quercetin (a natural bioflavonoids) 250 mg, Standardized Licorice root (13-15% glycyrrhizin) 600 mg, Selenium (selenomethionine) 100 mcg, in a synergistic base of White willow, odorless garlic, certified potency Bilberry (standardized for 25% anthocyanosides) and aromatic oil.

Adults take 3 capsules in the evening, preferably with meals.

Available in 30 capsules.

Internal use. Preservative-free.

Capsule.

Inflama-Force

Prairie Naturals®

Each 2 capsules contains: Curcumin (turmeric) (Curcuma longa) 350 mg, Bromelain (2000 mcu/g) 350 mg, L-Glutamine 300 mg, Glucosamine sulfate 200 mg, Yucca root powder (yucca spp.) 100 mg, organic Alfalfa leaf powder (Medicago sativa) 200 mg.

Take 2-4 capsules daily, between meals or as directed by a physician.

Available in 90 and 180 capsules.

Internal use. Contains no yeast, gluten, starch, egg, dairy, artificial color, preservatives, solvents, or alcohol.

Capsule.

Visual.

Inner Peace®
Penetrating Gel

Inno-Vite Inc.

Contains: Water, 8% extract of Mexican wild yam, 2% extract of Chaste tree berry, 2% extract of Chamomile, 2 % Vitamin E, Carbopol 934, Triethanolamine, Methyl paraben, Propyl paraben.

Apply twice daily for 3 weeks, massage 1/4 to 1/2 tsp. on the neck, wrists, breasts or inner arms. Alternate areas of application periodically.

Available in 60 g and 120 g.

External use.

Gel.

Do not apply during first seven days of menstrual cycle.

Visual.

Insure Herbal®

McZand® Herbal Inc.

Contains: Echinacea (E. Angustifolia root) and Goldenseal (Hydrastis canadensis root), in a base of Red clover blossom, Sage leaf, Burdock root, Peppermint leaf, Prairie dock root, Parsley leaf, Fennel seed, Ginger root, Elecampane root, Bayberry bark, Chamomile blossom, Scullcap herb, Valerian root, Barberry bark, Blessed thistle herb and Cayenne. Herbs extracted in distilled water, grain alcohol (ethyl alcohol USP) and vegetable glycerine. Contains 16-18% alcohol.

Take 20-40 drops or 2 tablets between meals 2-3 times daily.

Available in 30, 59, and 118 ml liquid and 50, 100 and 250 tablets.

Internal use.

Tablet.

Tincture.

Do not take if you have an auto-immune disease.

Ipecac
Homeopathic Remedy

A. Nelson & Company Ltd.

Each pillule contains: Ipecacuanha 6c.

Take 2 pillules every 2 hours for the first 6 doses, then 4 times daily for up to 5 days. Pillules should be sucked or chewed and taken between meals.

84 pillules/globules per bottle.

Internal use.

Pillule/globule.

Iron Chelated 25 mg

Natural Factors® Nutritional Products Ltd.

Each tablet contains: elemental Iron (HVP* chelate) 25 mg. *Hydrolyzed vegetable protein (sourced from rice).

Take 1 tablet daily or as directed by a physician.

Available in 90 tablets.

Internal use. Contains no artificial preservatives, color, dairy, sweeteners, starch, wheat or yeast.

Tablet.

There is enough iron in this product to seriously harm a child.
Visual.

Iron Plus

Natural Factors® Nutritional Products Ltd.

Each tablet contains: elemental Iron (Ferrous fumerate) 60 mg, Vitamin C 50 mg, elemental Manganese (Gluoconate) 2 mg, Vitamin B 12 (Cyanocobalamin) 10 mcg, Folic acid 0.1 mg. Non-medicinal ingredient: Dessicated liver powder 200 mg.

Take 1 tablet daily or as directed by a physician.

Available in 90 tablets.

Internal use. Contains no artificial preservatives, color, dairy, sweeteners, starch, wheat or yeast.

Tablet.

There is enough iron in this product to seriously harm a child.

Visual.

ISO3®
Complete Food

Next Nutrition

Contains: WPH - Whey peptides [modified molecular weight and partially predigested (hydrolyzed) Whey protein concentrate (providing di-, tri-, oligo and poly-peptides) (shorter and longer chains of amino acids)] and Ion-exchanged Whey, AmyloCarb™ [high molecular weight Amylopectin (modified food starch)], LipidLyte™ (structured lipid complex comprising high oleic Sunflower oil and Medium chain triglycerides), Whey glutamine peptide blend, Soy fiber, Chelatamin™ (chelated mineral transport blend comprising Calcium lactate, Zinc histidine, Zinc lactate, Iron histidine, Folic acid, Biotin, Chromium arginate, Chromium picolinate, Potassium iodide, Calcium phosphate, Sodium chloride, Copper histidine, Magnesium malate, Magnesium lactate, Magnesium pyruvate, Potassium phosphate), Vitamin E succinate, Vitamin D3, Vitamin A palmitate, Calcium ascorbate, Thiamine, Pyridoxine, Riboflavin, Calcium pantothenate, Cyanocobalamin, Inositol nicotinate, Lecithin, Vanilla flavor, Xanthan food gum, Vanilla extract, Acesulfame-k, Aspartame, Lactoperoxidase.

Add 3 scoops (72 g) to 12-16 oz. of liquid. Use ISO3 anytime throughout the day.

Available in 2.38 lbs.

Internal use.

Powder.

Visual.

Jade Immune Screen Powerful Defense® Capsules

Traditional Yin-Yang Herbals

Flora Manufacturing & Distributing Ltd.

Each capsule contains: Powered aqueous extracts of: Ban Ian gen (Isatidis seu baphicaccanthi, radix), Huang qi (Astragali membranacei, radix), Fang feng (Ledebouriellae divaricate,

radix), Bai zhu (Atractylodis macrocephalae, rhizoma), Nu zhen zi (ligustri lucidi, fructus), Ling zhi (Ganoderma lucidum), Gan cao (Glycyrrhizae uralensis, radix), Gui zhi (Cinnamomi cassiae, ramulus), Echinacea root; spray dried on a cornstarch carrier. 1:5 aqueous extract.

Take 2-3 capsules daily with liquid. Take with meals. For intense use: take 4 to 5 capsules daily. Take the capsules for 7 days. Stop for 2 days. Repeat cycle.

Available in 90 capsules of 450 mg in amber bottle.

Internal use. As presented by Dr. Malik Cotter (Diplomate of Oriental Medicine).

Vegetarian capsule.

Pregnant women should consult a physician before taking this formula.

Jade Immune Screen Powerful Defense® Tonic

Traditional Yin-Yang Herbals

Flora Manufacturing & Distributing Ltd.

Each 500 ml contains: Purified water; aqueous extracts of: Ban lan gen (Isatidis seu baphicaccanthi, radix), Huang qi (Astragali membranacei, radix), Fang feng (Ledebouriellae divaricate, radix), Bai zhu (Atracylodis macrocephalae, rhizoma), Nu zhen zi (Ligustri lucidi, fructus), Ling zhi (Ganoderma licidum), Gan cao (Glycyrrhizae uralensis, radix), Gui zhi (Cinnamomi cassiae, ramulus), Coneflower (Echinacea, radix).

Take 2 tbsp. 2-3 times daily with meals. For intense use: Take 3 tbsp. two to three times daily with meals. Dilute with warm water, if desired. Stop for two days. Repeat cycle.

Available in 500 ml amber bottle.

Internal use. No preservatives added. To prevent contamination do not drink directly from bottle and keep refrigerated after opening. Shelf life after opening is 14 days. As presented by Dr. Malik Cotter (Diplomate of Oriental Medicine).

Tonic.

Pregnant women should consult a physician before taking this formula.

Japanese Shark Cartilage Extract

22% Mucopolysaccharides

Natural Factors® Nutritional Products Ltd.

Each capsule contains: Shark cartilage extract powder 500 mg.

Take 1-3 capsules daily or as directed by a physicians.

Available in 90 and 180 capsules.

Internal use. Contains no artificial preservatives, color, dairy, sweeteners, starch, wheat or yeast. Natural factors shark cartilage is deodorized, filtered and sterilized into a purified, soluble powder that is then further processed to maximize its 22% mucopolysaccharide content.

▭ Capsule.

📷 Visual.

Jasmine Absolute
Essential Oil

🏠 **Bach-Karooch Ltd.**

⚗ Contains: Jasminum grandiflorum 100%.

✋ Two parts Essential oil must be diluted in 98 parts vegetable oil before applying to the skin. Consult Aromatherapy literature for specific methods of use and directions for each oil.

▣ 10 ml in amber bottle with child-resistant cap and one-drop insert.

◊ Oil.

⚠ Caution: due to high concentration, all oils may be harmful if improperly used!
External use only.

Joint Ease Formula

🏠 **Natural Factors® Nutritional Products Ltd.**

⚗ Each capsule contains: Devil's claw extract (3% Harpagosides) (Harpagophytum procumbens) 100 mg, Sarsaparilla root 4:1 extract (Smilax officinalis) 75 mg, Licorice extract (12% glycyrrhizin) (glycyrrhiza glabra) 50 mg, Yucca 4:1 extract (40% saponins) 50 mg, Alfalfa herb 5:1 extract (Medicago sativa) 25 mg, in a base of Flaxseed oil.

✋ Take 1-3 capsules daily.

90 softgel capsules.

🔢 Internal use. Contains no artificial preservatives, color, dairy, starch, wheat or yeast.

▭ Softgel capsule.

📷 Visual.

Juniper Berry
Essential Oil

🏠 **Bach-Karooch Ltd.**

⚗ Contains: Juniperus communis 100%.

✋ Two parts Essential oil must be diluted in 98 parts vegetable oil before applying to the skin. Consult Aromatherapy literature for specific methods of use and directions for each oil.

▣ 10 ml in amber bottle with child-resistant cap and one-drop insert.

◊ Oil.

⚠ Caution: due to high concentration, all oils may be harmful if improperly used!
External use only. Avoid during pregnancy.

Kali. Bich.
Homeopathic Remedy

🏠 **A. Nelson & Company Ltd.**

⚗ Each pillule contains: Kali bichromicum 6c.

✋ Take 2 pillules every 2 hours for the first 6 doses, then 4 times daily for up to 5 days. Pillules should be sucked or chewed and taken between meals.

84 pillules/globules per bottle.

🔢 Internal use.

⊘ Pillule/globule.

Kali. Phos.
Homeopathic Remedy

🏠 **A. Nelson & Company Ltd.**

⚗ Each pillule contains: Kali phosphoricum 6c.

✋ Take 2 pillules every 2 hours for the first 6 doses, then 4 times daily for up to 5 days. Pillules should be sucked or chewed and taken between meals.

▣ 84 pillules/globules per bottle.

🔢 Internal use.

⊘ Pillule/globule.

KAMA C.A.Z.E.
Vitamin C plus Zinc & Beta Carotene

🏠 **Albi Imports Ltd.**

⚗ Each tablet contains: Beta carotene 3200 IU, Vitamin C (Ascorbic acid and Zinc ascorbate) 200 mg, Zinc (ascorbate) 5 mg, Non-medicinal herbs: Echinacea augustifolia 6.5:1 (60 mg) 390 mg, Ginger 50 mg, Wild cherry bark 25 mg, Licorice 60 mg.

✋ Take 3 tablets daily, 1/2 dosage for children under 12.

▣ Available in 45, 90, 180 and 500 tablets/chewable lozenges and liquid, 125 ml and 250 ml.

Internal use.

Tablet.

Visual.

Kamut®

Artesian Acres Inc.

Contains: Whole Kamut® Grain.

Certified organic food. Kamut® is available as whole grain, flour and flakes, as well as breakfast cereals, pastas, Japanese noodles, breads, cookies, mixes etc. The International Allergy Association has found 74% of those with wheat sensitivities have little or no reaction to Kamut®.

Visual.

Kelp Alfalfa & Trace Minerals

Nutra Research International

Each capsule contains: Kelp, Alfalfa & Trace minerals 800 mg, Iodine 450 mcg. (from kelp).

Take 2 capsules daily with meals. 6 daily for therapeutic use.

120 capsules.

Provides the following minerals: Boron, Calcium, Chromium, Germanium, gold, Iodine, Iron, Magnesium, Manganese, Molybdenum, Phosphorus, Platinum, Potassium, Selenium, Silicon, Silver, Sodium, Vanadium, Zinc.

Capsule.

Kemi-Paste

Bio-Plex Products

Contains: White clay, Phosphates of Calcium/Sodium/Potassium/Iron/Magnesium, Fluoride of Calcium, Sulphate of Calcium/Sodium/Potassium, Potassium chloride, Silicon dioxide, essential oil of Lavender, Methyl paraben and glydant.

Apply an even coat on affected area and cover with a sterile cloth. Leave on overnight and remove in the morning with warm water.

100 cc

External use only. Not tested on animals.

Paste.

Kindervital Multivitamin for Children

Salus-Haus

Each tsp. (5 ml = 6 g) contains: Medicinal ingredients: Vitamin A 1250 IU, Vitamin D 100 IU, Calcium 50.1 mg (from Calcium gluconate and Calcium hypophosphite), Vitamin C 25 mg, Magnesium 7.25 mg (from Magnesium hydrogen phosphate), Vitamin E 6.25 IU, Niacinamide 2.5 mg, Thiamine 0.375 mg, Riboflavin 0.375 mg, Pyridoxine hydrochloride 0.375 mg, Cyanocobalamin 1.5 mcg, Folic acid 0.025 mg. Herbal ingredients: 2.16 g herb extract from: Carrots 21.6 mg, Anise seed 8.8 mg, Licorice root 6.4 mg, Milfoil herb 6.4 mg, Plantain herb 6.1 mg, Horsetail herb 6.0 mg, Camomile flowers 4.0 mg, Peppermint leaves 4.0 mg, Watercress 4.0 mg, Wheat germ 4.0 mg, Coriander seed 2.4 mg, Nettles 2.4 mg, Spinach 2.4 mg, Orange peel 1.6 mg. In a base of: Orange juice 0.8 g, Malt extract 0.431 g, Yeast extract 0.4 g, Pear juice concentrate 0.75 g, Maple syrup 0.375 g, Rosehip extract 0.145 g, Wheat germ extract 0.045 mg. Made up to 5 ml with natural corrigents.

Infants up to 1 year of age: 1 tsp. 1-2 times daily. Children under 6 years of age: 1 tsp. 2-3 times daily. Children over 6 years and young adults: 2 tsp. twice daily. Also suitable for adults. May be mixed with juice or distilled water.

Available in bottles of 10 ml trial size, 250 and 500 ml.

Internal use. Children's herbal multivitamin supplement.

Tonic.

KLB-5

Albi Imports Ltd.

Each tablet contains: Blue-green algae 100 mg, Bromelain 100 mg, Lecithin 100 mg, Kelp 100 mg, Apple cider vinegar 100 mg.

Take 2 tablets before each meal.

Available in 90 and 180 tablets.

Tablet.

Korean Ginseng Power Herb®

Nature's Herbs®

Each capsule contains: 100 mg certified potency® Korean white ginseng root extract concentrated and standardized for a minimum of the preferred 7% ginsenosides in a base of Wild countryside® Korean panax ginseng.

Adults take 1 capsule 2 times daily with a large glass of water.

Available in 50 capsules.

Internal use. Preservative-free.

Capsule.

Kyo-Dophilus®

Wakunaga of America Co., Ltd.

Each capsule contains: L. acidophilus, B. bifidum, and B. longum in a vegetable starch complex. 1.5 billion live cells at the time of shipment.

Take 1 capsule for adults (1/2 capsule for children under four) with a meal, twice daily.

Available in 45 capsules.

Internal use. Suitable for all ages. Milk-free and heat resistant. Free of preservatives, sugar, sodium, milk derivatives, yeast, gluten, artificial colors, flavors.

Capsule.

Visual.

Kyolic® Aged Garlic Extract™

Wakunaga of America Co., Ltd.

Each capsule contains: Aged Garlic extract powder 600 mg.

Take 2 capsules with a meal twice daily.

Available in 100 capsules.

Internal use.

Capsule.

Visual.

Kyolic Echinacea
With Aged Garlic Extract™

Wakunaga of America Co., Ltd.

Each capsule contains: Aged Garlic extract powder (Allium sativum) (bulb) 300 mg, Echinacea extract powder (Echinacea angustifolia) (root) 50 mg.

Take 2 capsules twice daily with meal.

Available in 100 capsules.

Internal use. The Echinacea in this formula is a 5:1 standardized extract and is equivalent to one gram of common dried root.

Capsule.

L-Glutamine
Amino Acid

Klaire Laboratories, Inc., USA & Europe

Each capsule contains: L-Glutamine 500 mg. Added ingredients: Cellulose & L-leucine.

Take 1 capsule daily or as directed by a physician.

Available in 100 capsules.

Internal use.

Capsule.

L-Tyrosine

Klaire Laboratories, Inc., USA & Europe

Each capsule contains: L-Tyrosine 500 mg. Added ingredient: L-leucine.

Take 1 capsule daily or as directed by a physician.

Available in 100 capsules.

Internal use.

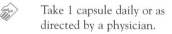

Capsule.

Larch
Bach Flower Remedy

🏠 **Bach Flower Remedies® Ltd.**

⚗ Contains: Larix decidua 5x in 27% grape alcohol solution.

✋ Take 2 drops under the tongue 4 times daily or 2 drops in a small glass of spring water and sip at intervals.

🧴 10 ml with dropper.

Ⅱ Internal use.

💧 Liquid.

Lavender
Essential Oil

🏠 **Bach-Karooch Ltd.**

⚗ Contains: Lavendula angustifolia 100%.

✋ Two parts Essential oil must be diluted in 98 parts vegetable oil before applying to the skin. Consult Aromatherapy literature for specific methods of use and directions for each oil.

🧴 10 ml in amber bottle with child-resistant cap and one-drop insert.

💧 Oil.

⚠ Caution: due to high concentration, all oils may be harmful if improperly used! External use only.

Lavilin Cream Body Deodorant
For Men and Women

🏠 **Lavilin™ Cosmetics**

⚗ Deodorant contains: Zinc oxide, Petroleum jelly, Talc, Potato starch, Calendula oil, Arnica oil, vitamin E, Ascorbyl palmitate, Citric acid, natural fragrance.

✋ One application can eliminate foot odor for days-no need to re-apply after bathing, exercise or strenuous activity.

🧴 0.44 oz.

Ⅱ Aluminum and alcohol-free. Not tested on animals.

🧴 Cream.

✋ If irritation occurs, discontinue use.

Lavilin Cream Foot Deodorant

🏠 **Lavilin™ Cosmetics**

⚗ Cream contains: Zinc oxide, Petroleum jelly, Talc, Potato starch, Calendula oil, Arnica oil, Vitamin E, Ascorbyl palmitate, Citric acid, natural fragrance.

✋ One application can eliminate foot odor for days. No need to re-apply after bathing, exercise or strenuous activity.

🧴 0.44 oz.

Ⅱ Aluminum and alcohol-free.

🧴 Cream.

✋ If irritation occurs, discontinue use.

Laxative Formula

🏠 **Natural Factors® Nutritional Products Ltd.**

⚗ Each capsule contains: Cascara Sagrada extract (50% cascarosides) (Rhamnus purshiana) 50 mg, Rhubarb root 4:1 extract (Rheum officinale) 25 mg, Cool Capsicum powder (Capsicum frutescens) 50 mg, Gentian root powder (Gentian lutea) 50 mg, Flax meal powder (Linum usitatissimum) 50 mg, Peppermint oil (Mentha piperita) 1.2 mg, in a gelatin capsule with cellulose.

✋ Take 1-3 capsules daily.

🧴 Available in 90 capsules.

Ⅱ Internal use. Contains no artificial preservatives, color, dairy, sweeteners, starch, wheat or yeast.

💊 Capsule.

📷 Visual.

LB Formula®

🏠 **Nature's Herbs®**

⚗ Each 434 mg capsule contains: Aged Cascara sagrada bark 95 mg. Other ingredients: Goldenseal root, Barberry bark, Ginger root, Red raspberry leaves, Rhubarb root, Fennel, Cayenne and Lobelia.

✋ Adults and children over 15 years of age: take 3-6 capsules before bedtime. Children 8 to under 15 take 1-2 capsules before bedtime, or as directed by a doctor.

Available in 100 capsules.

Internal use. Preservative-free.

Capsule.

Do not use laxative products when abdominal pain, nausea, or vomiting are present, or for a period longer than 1 week unless directed by a doctor.

Lemon
Essential Oil

Bach-Karooch Ltd.

Contains: Citrus limonum 100%.

Two parts Essential oil must be diluted in 98 parts vegetable oil before applying to the skin. Consult Aromatherapy literature for specific methods of use and directions for each oil.

10 ml in amber bottle with child-resistant cap and one-drop insert.

Oil.

May cause dermal irritation. Phototoxic on skin in direct sunlight.

Caution: due to high concentration, all oils may be harmful if improperly used! External use only.

Lemongrass
Essential Oil

Bach-Karooch Ltd.

Contains: Cymbopogen citratus 100%.

Two parts Essential oil must be diluted in 98 parts vegetable oil before applying to the skin. Consult Aromatherapy literature for specific methods of use and directions for each oil.

10 ml in amber bottle with child-resistant cap and one-drop insert.

Oil.

Possible skin irritant in some individuals.

Caution: due to high concentration, all oils may be harmful if improperly used! External use only.

Leritone Junior

Yves Ponroy

Each capsule contains: Cerebral phospholipids, Fish milt, Vitamin E and B12.

Adult or children: take 3 capsules daily for a minimum of 2 months.

Available in 60 capsules per box in blister packs.

Internal use.

Capsule.

Leritone Magnesium

Yves Ponroy

Each capsule contains: Vitamin E 2.75 IU, polyunsaturated long-chained cerebral phospholipids 22 mg.

Take 4 capsules daily for a minimum of 2 months.

Available in 60 capsules per box in blister packs.

Internal use.

Capsule.

Leritone Senior

Yves Ponroy

Each capsule contains: Medicinal ingredients: Vitamin C (dried acerola juice) 13 mg, Vitamin E (Vegetable oil concentrate) 6 IU, Selenium (Yeast) 24.5 mcg. Non medicinal: Oil from cold salt-water fish 265 mg, Citrus flavonoid compounds (peel of orange), 100 mg, Copra triglycerides 60 mg, Cerebro-extracts at 50%-30 mg, Carrot oleoresin 25 mg, Capsule: Gelatin, Glycerol, Water. Emulsifying agent: Soya bean lecithin.

Take 2 capsules daily for a minimum of 2 months.

Available in 40 capsules per box in blister packs.

Internal use.

Capsule.

LG Cleanse Formula

Natural Factors® Nutritional Products Ltd.

Each capsule contains: Milk thistle extract (10% Silymarin) (Silybum marianum) 100 mg, Turmeric extract (7-9% curmin) (Curcuma longa) 50 mg, Dandelion root 4:1 extract (Taraxacum officinale) 25 mg, Artichoke powder (Cynara scolymus) 100 mg, Celandine powder (Chelidonium majus) 5 mg, in a gelatin capsule.

Take 1-3 capsules daily.

Available in 90 capsules.

Internal use. Contains no artificial preservatives. color, dairy, sweeteners, starch, wheat or yeast.

Capsule.

Visual.

Licorice Phytosome

Nature's Herbs®

Each capsule contains: Licorice phytosome 100 mg (concentrated and standardized at 27-31% Glycyrrhetinic acid).

Take 2 capsules daily, preferably 1 with morning and evening meals.

Available in 60 softgel capsules.

Internal use.

Softgel capsule.

Do not take this product if you have heart disease or high blood pressure.

Licorice Root

Nature's Herbs®

Each 444 mg capsule contains: Wild countryside® Licorice root.

Take 3 capsules 3 times daily with a large glass of water.

Available in 100 capsules.

Internal use. Preservative-free.

Capsule.

Lime
Essential Oil

Bach-Karooch Ltd.

Contains: Citrus aurantifolia 100%.

Two parts Essential oil must be diluted in 98 parts vegetable oil before applying to the skin. Consult Aromatherapy literature for specific methods of use and directions for each oil.

10 ml in amber bottle with child-resistant cap and one-drop insert.

Oil.

May cause phototoxicity in some individuals.

Caution: due to high concentration, all oils may be harmful if improperly used!
External use only.

Liquid Calcium-Magnesium Citrate

Life-Time Nutrition Inc.

Each tbsp. contains: Calcium

(Citrate, Lactate, Gluconate) 600 mg, Magnesium (citrate) 300 mg, Vitamin D (Cholecalciferol) 400 IU. Base contains: Water, Citric acid, Fructose, Ascorbic acid, Natural orange or vanilla flavor.

Take 1 tbsp. (15 ml) daily or as directed by a health professional.

480 ml per bottle.

Liquid.

Visual.

Longevity Vital Life Energy Formula
Traditional Yin-Yang Herbals

Flora Manufacturing & Distributing Ltd.

Each 450 mg capsule contains: Powered aqueous extracts of: Huang qi (Astragali membranacei, radix), Shu di huang (Rehmanniae glutinosae conquitae, radix), He shou wu (polygoni multifori, radix), Tian men dong (Asparagi cochinchinensis, tuber), Fu ling (Poiae cocos, sclerotium), Nu zhen zi (Ligusti lucidi, fructus), Dang gui (Angelicae sinensis, radix), Gou qi zi (Lycii, fructus), Mai men dong (Ophiopogonis japonici, tuber), Wu wei zi (Schisandrae chinensis, fructus), Hong ren shen (Panax ginseng, radix), Ling zhi (Ganoderma lucidum), Gan cao (Glycyrrhizae uralensis, radix), Tian qi (Notoginseng, radix); spray dried on a cornstarch carrier. 1:5 aqueous extract.

Take 3-4 capsules daily with liquid. Take the capsules for 7 days. Stop for 2 days. Repeat cycle. Reduce the amount by half for children.

Available in 90 capsules of 450 mg each in an amber bottle.

Internal use. As presented by Dr. Malik Cotter (Diplomate of Oriental Medicine).

Vegetarian capsule.

Do not use when suffering from a cold, the flu, or when digestion is disrupted. Pregnant women should consult their physician before taking this formula.

Longevity Vital Life Energy Formula Tonic

Traditional Yin-Yang Herbals

Flora Manufacturing & Distributing Ltd.

Each 500 ml contains: Purified water; aqueous extracts of: Huang qi (Astragali membranacei, radix), Shu di huang (Rehmanniae glutinosae conquitae, radix), He shou wu (polygoni multifori, radix), Tian men dong (Asparagi cochinchinensis, tuber), Fu ling (Poiae cocos, sclerotium), Nu zhen zi (Ligusti lucidi, fructus), Dang gui (Angelicae sinensis, radix), Gou qi zi (Lycii, fructus), Mai men dong (Ophiopogonis japonici, tuber), Wu wei zi (Schisandrae chinensis, fructus), Hong ren shen (Panax ginseng, radix), Ling zhi (Ganoderma lucidum), Gan cao (Glycyrrhizae uralensis, radix), Tian qi (Notoginseng, radix).

Shake the bottle well before use. Take 2 tbsp. (30 ml) 2 to 3 times daily. Dilute with warm water, if desired. Take

the formula until the bottle is finished. Stop for two days. Repeat cycle. Reduce amounts by half for children. Shelf life after opening is 14 days.

Available in 500 ml, amber bottle.

Internal use. No preservatives added. To prevent contamination do not drink directly from the bottle. After opening, keep refrigerated at all times. As presented by Dr. Malik Cotter (Diplomate of Oriental Medicine).

Tonic.

Lycopodium

Homeopathic Remedy

A. Nelson & Company Ltd.

Each pillule contains: Lycopodium clavatum 6c.

Take 2 pillules every 2 hours for the first 6 doses, then 4 times daily for up to 5 days. Pillules should be sucked or chewed and taken between meals.

84 pillules/globules per bottle.

Internal use.

Pillule/globule.

Lysn-Force™

Prairie Naturals®

Each capsule contains: Vitamin C (Ascorbic acid, rutin rose hip and acerola)

166.67 mg, Citrus bioflavonoids 33.3 mg, Vitamin B1 (Thiamine HCL) 15 mg, Vitamin B6 (Pyridoxine) 15 mg, Vitamin B12 (Cobalamin concentrate) 333 mcg, Zinc (citrate) 5 mg. Non-medicinal ingredient base: Echinacea (root powder 4:1) 25 mg, Red clover (blossom) 15 mg, Goldenseal (root powder) 10 mg. Formulated in a specially filtered hydrolyzed vegetarian protein base rich in Lysine 333.3 mg.

Take 1-3 capsules daily.

Available in 90 and 180 capsules.

Internal use.

Capsule.

Visual.

M.N.P. For Women

naka Sales Ltd.

Each capsule contains: approx. 472 mg of the following herbs: Wild yam, Dong quai, Blue cohosh, Black cohosh, Blessed thistle, Shepperd's purse.

Take 1 capsule 3 times daily with each meal or as directed by a professional.

Available in 150 capsules.

Internal use.

Gelatin capsule.

Not to be taken during pregnancy.

Magnesium Citrate

150 mg

🏠 **Natural Factors®
Nutritional Products Ltd.**

⚗ Each capsule contains: elemental Magnesium (citrate) 150 mg.

✋ Take 1-3 capsules daily or as directed by a physician.

📦 Available in 90 capsules.

Ⓘ Internal use. Contains no artificial preservatives, color, dairy, sweeteners, starch, wheat or yeast.

💊 Capsule.

📷 Visual.

Magnesium Complex

🏠 **Klaire Laboratories, Inc.,
USA & Europe**

⚗ Each capsule contains: Magnesium (Glycinate) 100 mg. Added ingredient: L-leucine.

✋ Take 1 capsule 3 times daily or as directed by a physician.

📦 Available in 100 capsules.

Ⓘ Internal use.

💊 Capsule.

Mandarin

Essential Oil

🏠 **Bach-Karooch Ltd.**

⚗ Contains: Citrus reticulata 100%.

✋ Two parts Essential oil must be diluted in 98 parts vegetable oil before applying to the skin. Consult Aromatherapy literature for specific methods of use and directions for each oil.

📦 10 ml in amber bottle with child-resistant cap and one-drop insert.

💧 Oil.

👶 May cause phototoxicity in some individuals.

⚠ Caution: due to high concentration, all oils may be harmful if improperly used!
External use only.

Manganese Chelated

50 mg

🏠 **Natural Factors®
Nutritional Products Ltd.**

⚗ Each tablet contains: elemental Manganese (HVP* chelate) 50 mg. *Hydrolyzed vegetable protein (sourced from rice).

✋ Take 1 tablet daily or as directed by a physician.

📦 Available in 90 tablets.

Ⓘ Internal use. Contains no artificial preservatives, color, dairy, sweeteners, starch, wheat or yeast.

⊘ Tablet.

📷 Visual.

Marjoram

Essential Oil

🏠 **Bach-Karooch Ltd.**

⚗ Contains: Origanum majorana 100%.

✋ Two parts Essential oil must be diluted in 98 parts vegetable oil before applying to the skin. Consult Aromatherapy literature for specific methods of use and directions for each oil.

📦 10 ml in amber bottle with child-resistant cap and one-drop insert.

💧 Oil.

⚠ Caution: due to high concentration, all oils may be harmful if improperly used!
External use only. Avoid during pregnancy.

Medicinal Tea: Asthma

🏠 **Flora Manufacturing &
Distributing Ltd.**

⚗ Contains: Licorice root (Glycyrrhiza glabra) 360 mg, Coltsfoot leaves (Tussilago farfara) 265 mg, Fennel seed (Foeniculum vulgare) 190 mg, Nettle leaves (Urtica dioica) 190 mg, Plantain (Plantago lanceolata) 190 mg, Thyme herb (Thymus vulgaris) 155 mg, Silverweed herb (Potentilla anserina) 115 mg, Icelandic moss herb (Cetraria islandica) 95 mg, Camomile flowers (Matricaria recutita) 75 mg, Elecampane root (Inula helenium) 75 mg, Peony root (Paeonia officinalis) 75 mg, Primrose herb (Primula vulgaris) 75 mg, Poppy flower (Papaver rhoeas) 40 mg.

✋ Infuse 1 tea bag in one cup of boiling water. Allow the herbs to steep for at least 10 minutes. Adult dose: 1-2 cups of tea per day for 4 to 6 weeks once a year.

Available in box of 20 tea bags or 38 g bulk form.

Internal use.

Herbal Tea.

Those with impaired liver function should consult a qualified practitioner before taking. Not recommended for pregnant or lactating women.

Medicinal Tea: Biliv Tonic

🏠 **Flora Manufacturing & Distributing Ltd.**

Contains: Raspberry leaves (Rubus idaeus) 285 mg, Strawberry leaves (Fragaria vesca) 285 mg, Peppermint leaves (Mentha piperita) 210 mg, Fennel seed (Foeniculum vulgare) 135 mg, Hops (Humulus lupulus) 115 mg, Cinquefoil herb (Potentilla reptans) 95 mg, Flax seed (Linum usitatissimum) 95 mg, Knotgrass herb (Polygonum aviculare) 95 mg, Licorice root (Glycyrrhiza glabra) 95 mg, Linden flowers (Tilia officianalis) 95 mg, Oregon Grape root (Mahonia aquifolium) 95 mg, Woodruff herb (Galium odorata) 95 mg, Sweet everlasting herb (Gnaphalium obtusifolium) 75 mg, Daisy flowers (Bellis perennis) 40 mg, Sage leaves (Salvia officinalis) 35 mg, Senna (Cassia angustifolia) 35 mg, Poppy flowers (Papaver rhoeas) 20 mg.

Infuse 1 tea bag in one cup of boiling water. Allow the herbs to steep for at least 10 minutes. Adult dose: 1-3 cups of tea per day for 4 to 6 weeks.

Available in box of 20 tea bags or 38 g bulk form.

Internal use.

Herbal Tea.

Not recommended for pregnant or lactating women.

Medicinal Tea: Bronchial

🏠 **Flora Manufacturing & Distributing Ltd.**

Contains: Hollyhock flowers (Alcea rosea) 570 mg, Coltsfoot leaves (Tussilago farfara) 345 mg, Licorice root (Glycyrrhiza glabra) 285 mg, High mallow flowers (Malva sylvestris) 210 mg, Fennel seed (Foeniculum vulgare) 170 mg, Plantain leaves (Plantago psyllium) 170 mg, Primrose herb (Primula vulgaris) 75 mg, Calendula flowers (Calendula officinalis) 75 mg.

Infuse 1 tea bag in a cup of boiling water. Allow the herbs to steep for at least 10 minutes. Adult dose: 1-2 cups of tea per day taken for up to 6 weeks.

Available in box of 20 tea bags or 38 g bulk form.

Internal use.

Herbal Tea.

If cough persists or if condition recurs more than twice a year, consult a qualified practitioner. Not recommended for pregnant or lactating women or those with impaired liver function.

Medicinal Tea: Diulaxa

🏠 **Flora Manufacturing & Distributing Ltd.**

Contains: Nettle leaves (Urtica dioica) 475 mg, Dandelion leaves (Taraxacum officinale) 190 mg, Speedwell herb (Veronica officinalis) 155 mg, Birch leaves (Betula pendula) 135 mg, Senna pods (Cassia angustifolia) 135 mg, Blackberry leaves (Rubus fruticosus) 135 mg, Fennel seed (Foeniculum vulgare) 115 mg, Yarrow herb (Achillea millefolium) 115 mg, Calendula flowers (Calendula officinalis) 95 mg, Linden flowers (Tilia officinalis) 75 mg, Black elder berries (Sambucus nigra) 75 mg, Peony root (Paeonia officinalis) 55 mg, Poppy flowers (Papaver rhoeas) 55 mg, Sweet everlasting herb (Gnaphalium obtusifolium) 55 mg, Uva-ursi leaves (Arctostaphylos uva-ursi) 55 mg.

Infuse 1 tea bag in one cup of boiling water. Allow the herbs to steep for 10 minutes. Adult dose: 1-3 cups of tea per day for 4 to 6 weeks.

Available in box of 20 tea bags or 38 g bulk form.

Internal use.

Herbal Tea.

Not recommended for pregnant or lactating women.

Medicinal Tea: Flugrip

🏠 **Flora Manufacturing & Distributing Ltd.**

Contains: Linden flowers (Tilia officinalis) 475 mg, Rosehips (Rosa) 420 mg, Blackberry leaves (Rubus fruticosus) 380 mg, Black elder berries (Sambucus nigra) 285 mg, Black currant leaves (Ribes nigrum) 190 mg, Calendula flowers (Calendula officinalis) 95 mg, Sweet ever-lasting herb (Gnaphalium obtusifolium) 55 mg.

Infuse 1 tea bag in one cup of boiling water. Allow the herbs to steep for at least 10 minutes. Adult dose: 3-4 cups of tea per day.

Available in box of 20 tea bags or 38 g bulk form.

Internal use.

Herbal Tea.

Not recommended for pregnant or lactating women.

Medicinal Tea: For Women

Flora Manufacturing & Distributing Ltd.

Contains: Yarrow herb (Achillea millefolium) 380 mg, Lady's mantle herb (Alchemilla vulgaris) 285 mg, Cinquefoil herb (Potentilla reptans) 265 mg, Chamomile flowers (Matricaria recutita) 225 mg, Calendula flowers (Calendula officinalis) 210 mg, Lemon balm herb (Melissa officinalis) 210 mg, Rosemary leaves (Rosmarinus officinalis) 210 mg, High mallow flowers (Malva sylvestris) 115 mg.

Infuse 1 tea bag in one cup of boiling water. Allow the herbs to steep for at least 10 minutes. Adult dose: 1-3 cups of tea daily as needed.

Available in box of 20 tea bags or 38 g bulk form.

Internal use.

Herbal Tea.

Not recommended for pregnant or lactating women.

Medicinal Tea: Glandure

Flora Manufacturing & Distributing Ltd.

Contains: Peppermint leaves (Mentha piperita) 285 mg, Birch leaves (Betula pendula) 190 mg, Icelandic Moss herb (Cetraria islandica) 190 mg, Juniper berries (Juniperus communis) 190 mg, Sage leaves (Salvia officinalis) 190 mg, Yarrow herb (Achilla millefolium) 190 mg, Black walnut leaves (Juglans nigra) 95 mg, Couchgrass herb (Elytrigia repens) 95 mg, Lavender flowers (Lavandula officinalis) 95 mg, Licorice root (Glycyrrhiza glabra) 95 mg, Plantain leaves (Plantago lanceolata) 95 mg, Shepherd's purse herb (Capsella bursa-pastoris) 95 mg, Tormentil root (Potentilla erecta) 95 mg.

Infuse 1 tea bag in one cup of boiling water. Allow the herbs to steep for at least 10 minutes. Adult dose: 1-3 cups of tea per day for 4 to 6 weeks.

Available in box of 20 tea bags or 38 g bulk form.

Internal use.

Herbal Tea.

Not recommended for pregnant or lactating women.

Medicinal Tea: Hautex

Flora Manufacturing & Distributing Ltd.

Contains: Dandelion leaves (Taraxacum officinale) 380 mg, Juniper berries (Juniperus communis) 190 mg, Raspberry leaves (Rubus idaeus) 190 mg, Rosehips (Rosa canina) 190 mg, Speedwell herb (Veronica officinalis) 190 mg, Yarrow herb (Achillea millefolium) 190 mg, Birch leaves (Betula pendula) 95 mg, Buckbean leaves (Menyanthes trifoliata) 95 mg, Calendula flowers (Calendula officinalis) 95 mg, Echinacea root (Echinacea purpurea) 95 mg, Nettle leaves (Urtica dioica) 95 mg, Rosemary leaves (Rosmarinus officinalis) 95 mg.

Infuse 1 tea bag in one cup of boiling water. Allow the herbs to steep for at least 10 minutes. Adult dose: 1-3 cups of tea daily for 4 to 6 weeks.

Available in box of 20 tea bags or 38 g bulk form.

Internal use.

Herbal Tea.

Not recommended for pregnant or lactating women.

Medicinal Tea: Laxative

Flora Manufacturing & Distributing Ltd.

Contains: Senna leaves (Cassia angustifolia) 230 mg, Birch leaves (Betula pendula) 190 mg, Juniper berries (Juniperus communis) 190 mg,

Buckthorn bark (Rhamnus purshianus) 155 mg, Flax seed (Linum usitatissimum) 155 mg, Licorice root (Glycyrrhiza glabra) 150 mg, Acacia flowers (Acacia spp.) 115 mg, Peppermint leaves (Mentha piperita) 115 mg, Anise seed (Pimpinella anisum) 95 mg, Oregon Grape root (Mahonia aquifolium) 95 mg, Speedwell herb (Veronica officinalis) 95 mg, Yarrow herb (Achillea millefolium) 95 mg, Black elder berries (Sambucus nigra) 55 mg, Coriander seed (Coriandrum sativum) 55 mg, Peony root (Paeonia officinalis) 55 mg, Wild Plum bark (Prunus subcordata) 55 mg.

Infuse 1 tea bag in one cup of boiling water. Allow the herbs to steep for at least 10 minutes. Adult dose: 1-3 cups of tea per day as needed.

Available in box of 20 tea bags or 38 g bulk form.

Internal use.

Herbal Tea.

Not for prolonged use. Those with ulcers, ulcerative colitis, hemorrhoids or a serious bowel condition should consult a qualified practitioner before taking. Do not combine with other laxatives. Not recommended for pregnant or lactating women.

Medicinal Tea: Nerval Tonic

Flora Manufacturing & Distributing Ltd.

Contains: Blackberry leaves (Rubus fruticosus) 285 mg, High mallow flowers (Malva sylvestris) 285 mg, Heather flowers (Calluna vulgaris) 190 mg, Peppermint leaves (Mentha piperita) 190 mg, Rosemary leaves (Rosmarinus officinalis) 190 mg, Sage leaves (Salvia officinalis) 190 mg, Licorice root (Glycyrrhiza glabra) 115 mg, Calendula flowers (Calendula officinalis) 95 mg, Hops (Humulus lupulus) 95 mg, Lavender flowers (Lavandula angustifolia) 95 mg, Speedwell herb (Veronica officinalis) 95 mg, St. John's wort herb (Hypericum perforatum) 75 mg.

Infuse 1 tea bag in one cup of boiling water. Allow the herbs to steep for at least 10 minutes. Adult dose: 1-3 cups of tea daily as needed.

Available in box of 20 tea bags or 38 g bulk form.

Internal use.

Herbal Tea.

Not recommended for pregnant or lactating women.

Medicinal Tea: Reducing Tea

Flora Manufacturing & Distributing Ltd.

Contains: Strawberry leaves (Fragaria vesca) 285 mg, Dandelion root (Taraxacum officinale) 190 mg, Fucus leaves (Fucus vesiculosus) 190 mg, Uva-ursi leaves (Arctostaphylos uva-ursi) 190 mg, Winter savory herb (Satureja montana) 190 mg, Celery seed (Apium graveolens) 95 mg, Hibiscus flowers (Hibiscus sabdariffa) 95 mg, Lemon peel (Citrus limon) 95 mg, Linden flowers (Tilia officinalis) 95 mg, Sandalwood bark (Santalum album) 95 mg, Senna leaves (Cassia angustifolia) 95 mg, Senna pods (Cassia angustifolia) 95 mg.

Infuse 1 tea bag in one cup of boiling water. Allow the herbs to steep for at least 10 minutes. Adult dose: 1-3 cups of tea daily for 4 to 6 weeks.

Available in box of 20 tea bags or 38 g bulk form.

Internal use.

Herbal Tea.

This tea has mild laxative properties.

Do not combine with other laxatives. Those with serious kidney disorders or bowel obstruction should consult a qualified practitioner before taking. Not recommended for pregnant or lactating women. Not for prolonged use.

Medicinal Tea: Rheumadix

Flora Manufacturing & Distributing Ltd.

Contains: Birch leaves (Betula pendula) 230 mg, Juniper berries (Juniperus communis) 230 mg, Horsetail herb (Equisetum arvense) 170 mg, Bilberry leaves (Vaccinium myrtillus) 150 mg, Burdock root (Arctium lappa) 150 mg, Uva- ursi leaves (Arctostaphylos uva-ursi) 135 mg, Black currant leaves (Ribes nigrum) 95 mg, Linden flowers (Tilia officinalis) 95 mg, Nettle leaves (Urtica dioica) 95 mg, Sage leaves (Salvia officinalis) 95 mg, Calendula flowers (Calendula officinalis) 75 mg, Knotgrass herb (Polygonum aviculare) 75 mg, Wild plum bark (Prunus subcordata) 75 mg, Yarrow herb (Achillea millefolium) 75 mg, High mallow flowers (Malva sylvestris) 40 mg, Mullein leaves (Verbascum thapsus) 40 mg, Poppy flowers (Papaver rhoeas) 40 mg, Sunflower petals (Helianthus annuus) 35 mg.

Infuse 1 tea bag in one cup of boiling water. Allow the herbs to steep for at least 10 minutes. Adult dose: 1-3 cups of tea daily for 4-6 weeks.

Available in box of 20 tea bags or 38 g bulk form.

Internal use.

Herbal Tea.

Those with serious kidney disorders should consult a qualified practitioner before taking. Not recommended for pregnant or lactating women.

Medicinal Tea: Stomach

Flora Manufacturing & Distributing Ltd.

Contains: Daisy flowers (Bellis perennis) 325 mg, Black currant leaves (Ribes nigrum) 190 mg, Peppermint leaves (Mentha piperita) 190 mg, Strawberry leaves (Fragaria vesca) 190 mg, Caraway seed (Carum carvi) 95 mg, Chamomile flowers (Matricaria recutita) 95 mg, Coriander seed (Coriandrum sativum) 95 mg, Fennel seed (Foeniculum vulgare) 95 mg, Fenugreek seed (Trigonella foenum-graecum) 95 mg, Flax seed (Linum usitatissimum) 95 mg, Juniper berries (Juniperus communis) 95 mg, Sage leaves (Salvia officinalis) 95 mg,

Senna leaves (Cassia angustifolia) 95 mg, Calendula flowers (Calendula officinalis) 75 mg, High mallow flowers (Malva sylvestris) 75 mg.

Infuse 1 tea bag in one cup of boiling water. Allow the herbs to steep for at least 10 minutes. Adult dose: 1-3 cups of tea daily as needed.

Available in box of 20 tea bags or 38 g bulk form.

Internal use.

Herbal Tea.

Do not exceed maximum daily dose. Not for prolonged use. Not recommended for pregnant or lactating women.

Medicinal Tea: Uratonic

Flora Manufacturing & Distributing Ltd.

Contains: Cranberry fruit (Vaccinium macrocarpon) 360 mg, Uva-ursi leaves (Arctostaphylos uva-ursi) 270 mg, Birch leaves (Betula pendula) 155 mg, Juniper berries (Juniperus communis) 155 mg, Winter savory herb (Satureja montana) 115 mg, Parsley seed (Petroselinum crispum) 95 mg, Anise seed (Pimpinella anisum) 75 mg, Calendula flowers (Calendula officinalis) 75 mg, Heather flowers (Calluna vulgaris) 75 mg, Knotgrass herb (Polygonum aviculare) 75 mg, Linden flowers (Tilia officinalis) 75 mg, Peppermint leaves (Mentha piperita) 75 mg, Rose petals (Rosa sp.) 75 mg, Rupture wort herb (Herniaria glabra) 75 mg, Sweet everlasting herb (Gnaphalium obtusifolium) 75 mg, Yarrow herb (Achillea millefolium) 75 mg.

Infuse 1 tea bag in one cup of boiling water. Allow the herbs to steep for at least 10 minutes. Adult dose: 1 cup of tea four times daily.

Available in box of 20 tea bags or 38 g bulk form.

Internal use.

Herbal Tea.

Those with serious kidney disorders and those whose condition persists for more than 10 days should consult a qualified practitioner before taking. Not recommended for pregnant or lactating women.

Mega Acidophilus Powder with FOS
Non Dairy

Natural Factors® Nutritional Products Ltd.

Each 1/4 tsp. (1g) contains: 6 billion active cells of the following specially cultured strains of probiotics: L. rhamnosus 95% 5.70 billion, L. acidophilus 5% 0.30 billion bacteria to maintain healthful balance. FOS (Fructooligosaccharides: naturally occurring complex fructose molecules derived from chicory root) 200 mg. At time of manufacture guaranteed minimum 6 billion active cells per gram.

Take 1/4 tsp. at mealtime. Mix in juice, protein drinks or sprinkle on cereal or fruit.

Available in 75 g.

Internal use. No artificial preservatives, color, corn, dairy, soya, starch or yeast.

⟜ Powder.

📷 Visual.

🔲 Internal use.

▭ Capsule.

🔲 Internal use.

⊘ Tablet.

Mega Barley
Green Barley Extract

🏠 **Nutra Research International**

⚗ Contains: 100% Pure Barley extract powder.

👐 Take 1 1/2 tbsp. daily.

🗴 Available in 5.3 oz.

🔲 No added maltodextrins or additives. Organically grown on mineral rich soil.

⟜ Powder.

⚠ Lactating women.

Melbrosia® For Women

🏠 **Melbrosin International**

⚗ Each 460 mg capsule contains: Natural flower pollen (from 14 different plants), Beebread (fermented pollen), Royal jelly (lyophilized), Vitamin C (Acerola extract); in a pure gelatin capsule.

👐 For the first ten days, take 1 capsule 3 times daily before meals. For the next ten days, take 1 capsule twice daily before meals. Thereafter, take 1 capsule daily before meals. For best results, open capsule and dissolve contents in mouth before swallowing.

🗴 Available in 30 and 60 capsules, blisterpacked.

Melissa (RCO)
Essential Oil

🏠 **Bach-Karooch Ltd.**

⚗ Contains: Melissa officinalis 100%.

👐 Two parts Essential oil must be diluted in 98 parts vegetable oil before applying to the skin. Consult Aromatherapy literature for specific methods of use and directions for each oil.

🗴 10 ml in amber bottle with child-resistant cap and one-drop insert.

💧 Oil.

🤰 Possible sensitization and dermal irritation.

⚠ Caution: due to high concentration, all oils may be harmful if improperly used! External use only.

MENOPAUSE
Homeopathic Complex

🏠 **A. Nelson & Company Ltd.**

⚗ Each tablet contains: Sepia 6c, Pulsatilla 6c, Phosphorus 6c, Lachesis 6c, Actaea rac 6c.

👐 Suck or chew 2 tablets every 2 hours for 6 doses (12 tablets), then 2 tablets 3 times daily until symptoms subside.

🗴 72 tablets in blister packs.

Merc. Sol.
Homeopathic Remedy

🏠 **A. Nelson & Company Ltd.**

⚗ Each pillule contains: Mercurius solubilis hahnemanni 6c.

👐 Take 2 pillules every 2 hours for the first 6 doses, then 4 times daily for up to 5 days. Pillules should be sucked or chewed and taken between meals.

🗴 84 pillules/globules per bottle.

🔲 Internal use.

⊘ Pillule/globule.

Micel-A Micellized™ Vitamin A

🏠 **Klaire Laboratories, Inc., USA & Europe**

⚗ Each drop contains: 5,000 IU. Each dropper contains: 100,000 IU Micellized Vitamin A (Palmitate plus Beta carotene).

👐 Take 1 drop daily with food or juice or as directed by a physician.

🗴 Available in 1 fluid oz.

🔲 Internal use.

💧 Liquid.

Micel-E Micellized™ Vitamin E

🏠 **Klaire Laboratories, Inc., USA & Europe**

⚗️ Each dropper (1 ml) contains: 100 IU, Vitamin E as dl-alpha tocopheryl acetate in micellized form.

✋ Take 1 dropper (1 ml) daily with food or juice or as directed by a physician.

🗃️ Available in 1 fluid oz.

Ⓘ Internal use. Micellized™ for maximum absorption.

💧 Liquid.

Migra-Stress
Hi-Potency Feverfew

🏠 **Albi Imports Ltd.**

⚗️ Each capsule contains: Standardized organic feverfew leaf extract 250 mg of Fever leaf extract containing 0.5% Parthenolides.

✋ Take 1–2 capsules daily or as required.

🗃️ Available in 30, 60, 90 and 180 capsules.

Ⓘ Internal use.

💊 Capsule.

Migranon® Feverfew Extract

🏠 **Flora Manufacturing & Distributing Ltd.**

⚗️ Each 150 mg tablet contains: Medicinal ingredients: Standardized feverfew extract (Tanacetum parthenium) with a guaranteed minimum of 0.4 mg parthenolide.

✋ Take 1 tablet daily with water after meal. Consistent daily dosage is necessary to build and maintain therapeutic levels of parthenolide in the body.

🗃️ Available in amber bottle of 60 tablets.

Ⓘ Internal use.

⊘ Tablet.

⚠️ Do not use during pregnancy or lactation except on the advice of a physician.

Milk Thistle Phytosome™
150 mg

🏠 **Natural Factors® Nutritional Products Ltd.**

⚗️ Each capsule contains: Silymarin Phytosome™ (Silybum marianum) (Milk thistle extract bound to phosphatidyl choline from lecithin) 150 mg, standardized for flavonoid content of 80% Silymarin (120 mg), in a base of Dandelion, Artichoke and Turmeric. Encapsulated in a gelatin capsule with vegetable grade Magnesium stearate (used as a lubricant).

✋ Take 1-2 capsules at mealtime 3 times daily or as directed by a physician. Maximum daily dose 6 capsules.

🗃️ Available in 90 capsules.

Ⓘ Internal use. Contains no artificial preservatives, color, dairy, sweeteners, starch, wheat or yeast.

💊 Capsule.

📷 Visual.

Milk Thistle Power®

🏠 **Nature's Herbs®**

⚗️ Each capsule contains: 175 mg. Certified potency® Milk thistle extract concentrated and standardized for a minimum of preferred 80% Silymarin (140 mg per capsule), synergistically combined in a base of Turmeric and Artichoke.

✋ Take 1-2 capsules 3 times daily with water before meals.

🗃️ Available in 50 capsules.

Ⓘ Internal use. Preservative-free.

💊 Capsule.

Milk Thistle Tonic

🏠 **Anton Huebner GmbH & CO KG**

⚗️ Contains: Solid extract of Milk thistle fruit in a non-medicinal base of Sea buckthorn berry pulp, Fructose, Potassium sorbate and Vitamin C.

✋ Take 1 tbsp. 3 times daily after meals. Refrigerate after opening and shake well before use.

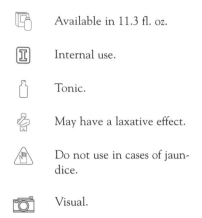

Available in 11.3 fl. oz.

Internal use.

Tonic.

May have a laxative effect.

Do not use in cases of jaundice.

Visual.

Mimulus
Bach Flower Remedy

Bach Flower Remedies® Ltd.

Contains: Mimulus guttatus 5x in 27% grape alcohol solution.

Take 2 drops under the tongue 4 times daily or 2 drops in a small glass of spring water and sip at intervals.

10 ml with dropper.

Internal use.

Liquid.

Mistletoe Tincture

Salus-Haus

Each 10 g tincture contains: 10 g extract derived from 2 g of Mistletoe plant.

Unless otherwise directed, take 15-20 drops diluted in a small amount of liquid 2-3 times daily.

Available in 50 ml, includes a dropper.

Internal use. Salus herbal tinctures are made in accordance with strictest health food principles, using natural ingredients only.

Tincture.

Mixed E 400 iu

Natural Factors® Nutritional Products Ltd.

Each capsule contains: 400 IU, of pure Vitamin E. in the form of d-alpha Tocopherol derived and isolated from 100% natural sources, plus additional mixed tocopherols Beta, Delta and Gamma in a balanced ratio. 100% Natural Source.

Take 1-2 capsules daily or as directed by a physician.

Available in 60, 90, 180 and 360 capsules.

Internal use. Contains no artificial preservatives, color, corn, dairy, gluten, starch or yeast.

Softgel capsule.

Visual.

Molkosan®
A. Vogel

Bioforce AG

Contains: Concentrated lactofermented whey without protein, (L+) Lactic acid.

Internally: take 1 tsp. to a glass of water. Externally: 1 part Molkoson in 4 parts water and rinse. Insect bites: apply undiluted on bite.

Available in 200 ml and 500 ml.

Internal and external use. Because of its acid pH value, Molkosan is recommended externally as a disinfectant.

Liquid.

Moonshine Silica Recovery Emollient

Prairie Naturals®

Contains: Silicon Dioxide (Silica 3% Volume) Trimethicone (Silica Extract), Vegetable Glycerine, Panthenol, Aloe Vera, Tocopherol, Natural Aromatic Oils of Geranium and Lemon, Rice Bran Oil, Methoxycinnamate, Grapefruit Seed Extract.

Apply 5-10 drops to damaged hair after washing and conditioning the hair. Do not rinse out. Style as usual.

Available in 125 ml dropper bottles.

External use only. Enviro-wise and biodegradable. Not tested on animals.

Liquid.

Multi Acidophilus
Non-Dairy

Natural Factors® Nutritional Products Ltd.

Each capsule contains: 4 billion active cells of the following specially cultured strains of probiotics: L. rhamnosus R011 35% 1.40 billion, E. faecium 20% 0.80 billion, B. longum 13.3% 0.53 billion, S. thermophilus 13% 0.52 billion, L. acidophilus 10% 0.40 billion, L. rhamnosus R049 6.7% 0.27 billion, L. delbrueckii subsp. bulgaricus 2% 0.08 billion. FOS (Fructooligosaccharides: naturally occurring complex fructose molecules derived from chicory root) 200 mg.

Take 3 capsules daily at mealtime.

Available in 60 and 90 capsules.

Internal use. Contains no artificial preservatives, color, corn, dairy, soya, starch or yeast. At time of manufacture guaranteed minimum 4 billion active cells per capsule.

Capsule.

Visual.

Multi-Element Buffered Vitamin C

Klaire Laboratories, Inc., USA & Europe

Each capsule contains: Vitamin C (Ascorbic acid, Potassium ascorbate, Calcium ascorbate, Magnesium ascorbate) 600 mg, Calcium (Carbonate, Ascorbate) 40 mg, Quercetin 30 mg, Magnesium (Carbonate, Ascorbate) 27 mg, Potassium (Ascorbate) 9 mg, Reduced L-Glutathione 5.9 mg, Zinc (Citrate) 3.2 mg, Manganese (Glycinate) 0.5 mg, Copper (Glycinate) 0.23 mg. Added ingredients: L-leucine and L-valine.

Take 2 capsules in the morning and 2 in the evening or as directed by a physician.

Available in 100 and 250 capsules.

All quantities of mineral are elemental.

Capsules.

Multi-Force™
Vitamin & Mineral Supplement

Prairie Naturals®

Each capsule contains: Beta carotene (Provitamin A) 2,500 IU, Vitamin A (Palmitate) 2,500 IU, Vitamin D (Cholecalciferol) 133.33 IU, Vitamin E (d-alpha Tocopheryl succinate) 133.33 IU, Vitamin C (Ascorbic acid) 133.33 mg, Vitamin B1 (Thiamine) 10 mg, Vitamin B2 (Riboflavin) 10 mg, Vitamin B3 (Niacinamide) 10 mg, Vitamin B6 (Pyridoxine hydrochloride) 10 mg, Vitamin B12 (Cobalamine) 33.3 mcg, Biotin 55 mcg, Folic acid (Folacin) 300 mcg, Pantothenic acid (Calcium d-pantothenate) 10 mg. Lipotropic factors: Choline (Bitartrate) 10 mg, Inositol 10 mg, DL-Methionine 10 mg. Minerals: Calcium (carbonate/citrate) 30 mg, Iron (Ferrous Fumarate) 5 mg, Magnesium (oxide/citrate) 30 mg, Zinc (citrate) 5 mg, Iodine (Potassium iodide) 0.1 mg, Manganese (gluconate/citrate) 2 mg, Copper (HVP* chelate) 1 mg, Chromium (amino acid chelate) 67 mcg, Selenium (amino acid chelate) 67 mcg, Vanadium (amino acid chelate) 25 mcg, Molybdenum (amino acid chelate) 17 mcg in a greenfood base of: Green tea extract (20% polyphenols)

30 mg, Alfalfa powder 10 mg, Royal jelly 10 mg, Siberian ginseng 10 mg, organic Carrot powder 10 mg, Spirulina (Blue green algae) 10 mg, Norwegian kelp powder 5 mg. Non-medicinal ingredients: Bromelain (2000 mcu/g) 10 mg, Papain 10 mg, Betaine HCL 10 mg, PABA (Para aminobenzoic acid) 5 mg, Citrus bioflavonoids 15 mg. *Hydrolyzed vegetable protein.

Take 3 capsules daily, 1 with each meal.

Available in 90, 180 and 360 capsules.

Internal use.

Capsule.

Visual.

Muscle & Joint Formula

Natural Factors® Nutritional Products Ltd.

Each capsule contains: Licorice extract (12% glycyrrhizin) (glycyrrhiza glabra) 100 mg, Chamomile 4:1 extract (anthemis nobilis) 50 mg, Marshmallow root 4:1 extract (althaea officinalis) 25 mg, Black Cohosh 4:1 extract (Cimicifuga racemosa) 25 mg, Turmeric (curcuma longa) 25 mg, Bromelain 1000 GDU 100 mg, in a gelatin capsule with rice protein.

Take 1-3 capsules daily.

Available in 90 capsules.

Internal use. Contains no artificial preservatives, color, dairy, sweeteners, starch, wheat or yeast.

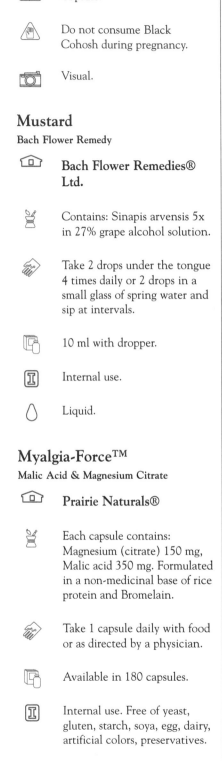

Capsule.

Do not consume Black Cohosh during pregnancy.

Visual.

Mustard
Bach Flower Remedy

🏠 **Bach Flower Remedies® Ltd.**

Contains: Sinapis arvensis 5x in 27% grape alcohol solution.

Take 2 drops under the tongue 4 times daily or 2 drops in a small glass of spring water and sip at intervals.

10 ml with dropper.

Internal use.

Liquid.

Myalgia-Force™
Malic Acid & Magnesium Citrate

🏠 **Prairie Naturals®**

Each capsule contains: Magnesium (citrate) 150 mg, Malic acid 350 mg. Formulated in a non-medicinal base of rice protein and Bromelain.

Take 1 capsule daily with food or as directed by a physician.

Available in 180 capsules.

Internal use. Free of yeast, gluten, starch, soya, egg, dairy, artificial colors, preservatives.

Capsule.

Visual.

Myrrh
Essential Oil

🏠 **Bach-Karooch Ltd.**

Contains: Commiphora myrrha 100%.

Two parts Essential oil must be diluted in 98 parts vegetable oil before applying to the skin. Consult Aromatherapy literature for specific methods of use and directions for each oil.

10 ml in amber bottle with child-resistant cap and one-drop insert.

Oil.

Caution: due to high concentration, all oils may be harmful if improperly used!
External use only. Avoid during pregnancy.

Myrtle
Essential Oil

🏠 **Bach-Karooch Ltd.**

Contains: Myrtus communis 100%.

Two parts Essential oil must be diluted in 98 parts vegetable oil before applying to the skin. Consult Aromatherapy literature for specific methods of use and directions for each oil.

10 ml in amber bottle with child-resistant cap and one-drop insert.

Oil.

Caution: due to high concentration, all oils may be harmful if improperly used!
External use only.

N-Acetyl L-Carnitine

🏠 **Klaire Laboratories, Inc., USA & Europe**

Each capsule contains: N-Acetyl L-Carnitine 250 mg. Added ingredient: L-leucine.

Take 1 or 2 capsules, 2 to 3 times daily, or as directed by a physician.

Available in 100 capsules.

Internal use. N-Acetyl L-Carnitine (NAC) is a naturally occurring Acetyl metabolite of the amino acid Carnitine.

Capsule.

NAG
N-Acetyl Glucosamine

🏠 **Quest Vitamins**

Each capsule contains: N-Acetyl glucosamine (NAG) 500 mg, Magnesium stearate (vegetable source), Capsule shell: Gelatin, Water.

Take 4 to 6 capsules daily.

Available in 500 mg; 60 and 90 capsules and 1000 mg; 60 tablets.

Internal use. Contains no artificial preservatives, colors, flavors or added sugar, starch, milk products, wheat or yeast.

Capsule.

Tablet.

Nat. Mur.
Homeopathic Remedy

🏠 **A. Nelson & Company Ltd.**

⚗️ Each pillule contains: Natrum muriaticum 6c.

🤚 Take 2 pillules every 2 hours for the first 6 doses, then 4 times daily for up to 5 days. Pillules should be sucked or chewed and taken between meals.

📦 84 pillules/globules per bottle.

Ⅱ Internal use.

⊘ Pillule/globule.

Natracare Feminine Hygiene®

🏠 **Bodywise (UK) Ltd.**

⚗️ Tampons are made from 100% cotton with biodegradable applicator. Panty shields are made from 100% fluff pulp. Pads are made from 100% fluff pulp with an additional plastic liner.

🤚 Use as required.

📦 All products (pads, tampons, panty shields) are packaged in recycled paper boxes - biodegradable.

Ⅱ Internal and external use. A complete line of non-chlorine bleached, disposable feminine hygiene products. All products are free of dioxins and additives.

Natural Lips
Crystal Clear Lip Gloss

🏠 **Aubrey Organics®**

⚗️ Contains: Essential fatty acid base, sunflower oil, Jojoba oil, Jojoba butter, Jojoba wax, PABA, African butter, Vitamin E and peppermint.

🤚 Apply to lips as needed.

📦 Available in 4 g.

Ⅱ Crystal clear shade. External use only. Also available in 3 shades: natural red, petal pink and mocha brown. No artificial additives. SPF 15 sun protection.

Natural Resources MELATONIN

🏠 **Scandinavian Natural Health & Beauty Products. Inc.**

⚗️ Each tablet contains: Melatonin 3 mg, Vitamin B6 1 mg. Each sublingual tablet contains: Melanin 2-5 mg, Coenzyme Vitamin B6 500 mcg.

🤚 Take regular tablets: 1-2 tablets 1-2 hours before bedtime. Sublingual: 1-2 tablets 12-20 minutes before bedtime.

📦 Available in 30, 60, and 120 tablets (regular) and 120 sublingual tablets.

Ⅱ Internal use. Flavored sublingual tablets contain natural orange or natural peppermint flavor.

⊘ Tablet and sublingual tablet.

⚠️ Recommended dosages for temporary use. Melatonin should not be used by children, pregnant or lactating women, by people taking steroid drugs such as cortisone or by people with an over active immune system (autoimmune diseases, lymphoma, leukemia)

Neroli
Essential Oil

🏠 **Bach-Karooch Ltd.**

⚗️ Contains: Citrus aurantium 100%.

🤚 Two parts Essential oil must be diluted in 98 parts vegetable oil before applying to the skin. Consult Aromatherapy literature for specific methods of use and directions for each oil.

📦 10 ml in amber bottle with child-resistant cap and one-drop insert.

💧 Oil.

⚠️ Caution: due to high concentration, all oils may be harmful if improperly used! External use only.

Nerve & Stress Formula

🏠 **Natural Factors® Nutritional Products Ltd.**

⚗️ Each capsule contains: St. John's wort extract (0.3% hypericin) (Hypericum perforatum) 100 mg, Kava-Kava 4:1 extract (Piper methysticum) 50 mg, Valerian 4:1 extract (Valeriana officinalis) 25 mg, Passion flower powder

(Passiflora incarnata) 100 mg, in a gelatin capsule with rice protein.

Take 1-3 capsules daily.

Available in 90 capsules.

Internal use. Contains no artificial preservatives, color, dairy, sweeteners, starch, wheat or yeast.

Capsule.

Visual.

Nettle Juice

W. Schoenenberger

Contains: Pure natural pressed herb and plant juice from organically grown Nettle plants.

Shake bottle before use. Take 3 or 4 times daily before meals 1 tbsp. diluted in water, milk or tea, one part juice to six parts liquid. For children 1 tsp. full instead of tbsp. Unopened bottle will keep indefinitely: opened, for 6 days.

Amber bottle of 5.5 fl. oz.

Internal use. Organically grown in nearly ideal conditions in the Black Forest & Swabian uplands, where the air is pure. The plants are gathered at the moment when their production of valuable ingredients is at its peak. The juices are extracted by specially designed hydraulic presses that ensure maximum recovery of all essential elements, making certain that not more than 2-3 hours elapse between harvesting, pressing and bottling.

Cellular plant juice.

Nettle Leaf

Nature's Herbs®

Each 480 mg capsule contains: Nettle leaf.

Take 1-2 capsules 2-3 times a day.

Available in 100 capsules.

Internal use. Preservative-free.

Capsule.

New Zealand Shark Cartilage

Natural Factors® Nutritional Products Ltd.

Each capsule contains: Shark cartilage extract powder 750 mg, in a gelatin capsule with microcrystalline cellulose.

Take 1-3 capsules daily or as directed by a physician.

Available in 90, 180 and 360 capsules.

Internal use. Contains no artificial preservatives, color, dairy, sweeteners, starch, wheat or yeast. Natural Factors shark cartilage is deodorized, filtered and sterilized into a purified, soluble powder. 18% Mucopolysaccharides.

Capsule.

Shark cartilage is not recommended for small children, pregnant or lactating women or recent heart attack sufferers.

Visual.

Niaouli
Essential Oil

Bach-Karooch Ltd.

Contains: Melaleuca viridiflora 100%.

Two parts Essential oil must be diluted in 98 parts vegetable oil before applying to the skin. Consult Aromatherapy literature for specific methods of use and directions for each oil.

10 ml in amber bottle with child-resistant cap and one-drop insert.

Oil.

Caution: due to high concentration, all oils may be harmful if improperly used! External use only.

NOCTURA™
Homeopathic Complex

A. Nelson & Company Ltd.

Each tablet contains: Kali brom 6c, Coffea 6c, Passiflora 6c, Avena sativa 6c, Alfalfa 6c, Valeriana 6c.

Take 2 tablets 4 hours before retiring. Repeat immediately before retiring. An additional 2 tablets may be taken during the night if required. Tablets should be dissolved in mouth or chewed. Take between meals.

72 tablets in blister packs.

Internal use.

Tablet.

If symptoms persist, consult a registered medical practitioner.

Norwegian Kelp

Nature's Herbs®

Each 646 mg capsule contains: Premium Norwegian sea kelp.

Take 1 capsule 3 times daily with a full glass of water.

Available in 100 capsules.

Internal use. Preservative-free.

Capsule.

Norwegian Kelp Combination

Nature's Herbs®

Each capsule contains: Vegetal plant source Iodine and trace minerals in varying amounts as naturally occur in Norwegian kelp, Irish moss, Cayenne and Parsley leaves and root.

Take 1-2 capsules 3 times daily with water.

Available in 100 capsules.

Internal use. Preservative-free.

Capsule.

Nova Depression Complex

Nova® Homeopathic Therapeutics Inc.

Contains: Antimonium crudum 12C, Calcarea carbonica 12C, Capsicum annum 12C, Kali phosphoricum 12C, Natrum muriaticum 12C, Phosforicum acidum 12C, Pulsatilla 12C, Rhus toxicodendron 12C, 20% USP Alcohol, a.a.

Adults: 12-15 drops 4-6 times daily, in acute phase every half hour until relief occurs; Children 2-12 years: 8-10 drops. Take directly under tongue or add to water.

Available in 1.7 oz.

Internal use.

Liquid.

Nova Lower Back Complex

Nova® Homeopathic Therapeutics Inc.

Contains: Causticum 6x, Colocynthis 4x, Rhus toxicodendrum 12x, Gnaphaliym poly. 6x, Ledum 6x, Berberis 4x, Ammonium mur. 8x, Phytolacca 6x, Stannum met. 8x, Apis 4x, Chelidonium 4x, Cuprum acet. 4x, 20% USP Alcohol, a.a. 8.33%.

Adults: 12-15 drops 4-6 times daily, in an acute phase; every half hour until relief occurs; Children 2-12 years: 8-10 drops. Take directly under tongue or add to water.

Available in 1.7 oz.

Internal use.

Liquid.

Nova Sinus Complex

Nova® Homeopathic Therapeutics Inc.

Contains: Antimonium tartaricum 6x, Bryonia 4x, Echinacea angustifolia 4x, Euphorbium officinarum 6x, Hepar sulphuris calcareum 8x, Hepatica tribola 4x, Hydrastis canadensis 4x, Natrum muriaticum 12x, Phosphorus 12x, 20% USP Alcohol, a.a.

Adults: 12-15 drops 4-6 times daily, in acute phase every half hour until relief occurs; Children 2-12 years: 8-10 drops. Take directly under tongue or add to water.

Available in 1.7 oz.

Internal use.

Liquid.

Nozovent®
Anti-Snoring Device

Scandinavian Natural Health & Beauty Products, Inc.

Anti-snoring device made of nontoxic, pharmaceutical grade plastic, approved by the FDA.

Device, simple to use.

Available in packages of one or two devices.

External use. Developed by a Swedish ENT physician. Enhances easy breathing, eliminates stuffy nose from colds and allergies, reduces or eliminates snoring, reduces sleep apnea, improves sleep. Nozovent increases the air flow through the nose by dilating the nostrils. Nozovent is reusable and washable for up to 3 months. Does not cause skin irritation.

NSR Natural Sports Rub

Warm up/Rub-Down Massage Lotion for Active People

Aubrey Organics®

Contains: Aubrey's natural fatty acid cream base contains oil of Wintergreen, oil of Rosemary, oil of cinnamon, oil of Ginger root, Vegetable glycerine, oil of Eucalyptus, Menthol, oil of Sage, Citrus seed extract, Vitamins C and E.

Apply before and after workouts.

Available in 4 fl. oz.

External use only. Vegan.

Lotion.

Nu-Body Advanced® 1000 mg Citrimax™

Nu-Life Nutrition Ltd.™

Each caplet contains: Chromium (amino acid chelate) 165 mcg. Non-medicinal ingredients: Garcinia cambogia 1000 mg supplying (-) Hydroxycitric acid (HCA) 500 mg in a base of Siberian ginseng, Cayenne and Gymnema sylvestre.

Take 1 caplet 1/2 hour before each meal (total 3 daily), or as directed by a health professional.

Available in 500 mg and 1000 mg, 90 caplets.

Internal use. Citrimax™ is derived from the dried rind of Garcinia cambogia, a native fruit of India.

Caplet.

Visual.

Nu-Greens® Profile

51 Functional Nutrients

Nu-Life Nutrition Ltd.™

Each 8.5 g contains: Pure soy lecithin 99% oil free (Essential fatty acids 538 mg, Phosphatidylcholine 469 mg, Phosphatidlylethanolamine 408 mg, Phosphatidylserine 300 mg, Phosphatidylinositol 285 mg) 2000 mg, Enzyme active 10:1 concentrates (Alfalfa grass juice powder, Barley greens juice powder, Buckwheat grass juice powder, Kamut cereal grass juice powder, Red beet juice powder, Wheat cereal grass juice powder) 1600 mg, Hawaiian Spirulina pacifica 1500 mg, Five-Fibre blend (Apple pectin fibre, Beet fibre, Carrot fibre, Oat fibre, Soy bran fibre) 1000 mg, Tomato powder (source of lycopene) 100 mg, Whole brown rice powder 500 mg, Sprouted multi-grains (Organic soybean sprouts, Barley malt sprouts, Wheat berry sprouts, Mung bean sprouts) 400 mg, Multi-Algae blend (Chlorella green algae, (cracked cell wall), Dunaliella salina red algae, Haematococcus pluvialis red algae (source of astaxanthin),

Kombu seaweed, Nova Scotia dulse, Phlorotannin extract of Canary Island brown algae, Wakame seaweed) 400 mg, Non-dairy eight culture multi strain probiotic blend (provides 2.5 billion organisms), (Lactobacillus acidophilus, Lactobacillus rhamnosus, Lactobacillus plantarum, Lactobacillus sporogenes, Lactobacillus salivarius, Lactobacillus caucasicus, Bifidobacterium longum, Bifidobacterium bifidum) 250 mg, FOS (fructo-oligosaccharides) (Dahlia, Dahlulin PB Probiotic Inulin, Chicory, Jerusalem artichoke) 250 mg, Royal jelly (from lyophilized 3.5:1 concentrate) 150 mg, Multi-floral wildflower Bee pollen 150 mg, Acerola berry juice powder 4:1 extract 125 mg, Milk thistle extract 30:1 60 mg, Licorice root Standardized extract (15% glycyrrhizin) 125 mg, Siberian ginseng root standardized extract (0.5% eleutherosides) 75 mg, Ginkgo biloba standardized extract 50:1 (24% ginkgo flavonglycosides, 6% terpene lactones) 20 mg, Non-fermented green tea standardized extract (60% polyphenols) 2000:1 15 mg, European bilberry standardized extract (25% anthocyanosides) 50:1 10 mg, Grape seed extract (95% proanthocyanidins) 60:1 5 mg, Astragalus root 50 mg, Stevia leaf standardized extract (85% steviosides) 5 mg.

Place one scoopful into a container, add 8 oz. of water or juice, mix well and drink.

Available in 255 g powder.

Internal use.

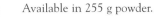
Powder.

Visual.

Nu-Greens® Prolong

Nu-Life Nutrition Ltd.™

Each capsule contains: Grape seed extract (ActiVin™) 75 mg, Resveratrol (proantho-cyanidins (95% activity), polyphenols (min. 46% activity), anthocyanidins (min. 30% activity), catechins (min. 18% activity) 15 mcg, Lipoic acid 12.5 mg, Beta carotene (natural carotenoids) 1500 IU, in a base of rice powder.

Take 1 capsule with breakfast and 1 with dinner.

60 capsules.

Capsule.

Visual.

Nu-Greens® Promote

Nu-Life Nutrition Ltd.™

Each 3 tsp. contains: High pectin multi fruit fiber (High pectin apple fiber, Citrus pectin cellulose complex, Prune fiber, Scandinavian beet fiber, Black currant fiber) 1750 mg, Whole leaf aloe vera gel (from lyophylized 200X concentrate equal to 30 g of whole leaf) 150 mg, Vegetable powder concentrate 10:1 (cruciferous and allium vegetables (source of indole-3-carbinol): Broccoli, Cauliflower, Cabbage, Kale, Leek, Onion, Garlic, Mustard greens. Carotenoid vegetables (supplies Beta carotene): Banana pepper, Carrot, Yellow squash, Yam. Leafy greens (source of chlorophyll): Parsley, Spinach, Amaranth, Watercress) 1000 mg, Organic cereal grasses (Flax meal, Alfalfa grass, Barley grass, Wheat grass, Oat bran, Tritacale greens) 2500 mg, Sprouted barley malt 500 mg, Brown rice solids 500 mg, Echinacea purpurea 500 mg, Probiotic support medium (Fructo-oligosaccharides (FOS) from Dahlia, Chicory, Jerusalem artichoke, Vegetable mannin oligo-saccharides (MOS), Caprylic acid) 1000 mg, Soy sprouts, organically grown 200 mg, Non-dairy eight culture multi strain probiotic blend (provides 2.5 billion organisms) (Lactobacillus acidophilus, Lactobacillus rhamnosus, Lactobacillus plantarum, Lactobacillus sporogenes, Lactobacillus salivarius, Lactobacillus caucasicus, Bifidobacterium longum, Bifidobacterium bifidum) 250 mg, Hawaiian Spirulina pacifica 200 mg, Full spectrum enzymes (Starch digesting enzymes: Alpha amylase, Beta amylase, Glucoamylase, Lactase, Maltase, Saccharase). Fat digesting enzymes: Esterase, Lipase, Lipoprotease. Fiber digesting enzymes: Cellullase, Hemicellulase, Pectinase. Protein digesting enzymes: Bromelain, Acid protease, Neutral peptidase, Papain. Total enzyme units 94330, Stevia leaf standardized extract (85% steviosides) 5 mg.

Place one scoopful into a container, add 8 oz. of water or juice, mix well and drink. Take at bedtime. Drink 8 glasses of liquids daily to help insure healthy intestinal function.

Available in 264 g powder.

Powder.

Visual.

Nu-Medicine® Cold/Flu
Homeopathic Remedy

Nu-Life Nutrition Ltd.™

Contains: Eucalyptus globulus 8x, Allium cepa 6x, Euphrasia 6x, Natrum muriaticum 10x, Sticta pulmonaria 8x, Gelsemium sempervirens 8x.

Take 3 granules at a time, 3 times daily, or as directed by a homeopathic practitioner.

120 granules.

Internal use.

Granules.

Nu-Medicine® Cough Syrup
Homeopathic Medicine

Nu-Life Nutrition Ltd.™

Contains: Belladonna 6x, Camphora 3x, Castanea vesca 2x, Hedera helix 4x, Hedera helix 8x, Hedera helix 12x, Senega 4x, Sticta pulmonaria 4x, Sticta pulmonaria 8x, Sticta pulmonaria 12x.

Take 2 tsp. 3-4 times daily, or as directed by a homeopathic practitioner.

200 ml.

Internal use.

Liquid.

Visual.

Nu-Source® Energin®
Enhanced Standardized Ginseng Phytosome

Nu-Life Nutrition Ltd.™

Each caplet contains: Multi-Ginseng standardized extract (10 mg ginsenosides) (Chinese ginseng root (Panax ginseng)/Red Korean Panax ginseng root (Panax ginseng)/Siberian ginseng root (Eleutherococcus senticosus)/Brazilian Ginseng root (Pfaffia paniculata)/Indian Ginseng root (Withania somnifera)/Canadian ginseng root (Panax quinquefolius)/Tienchi Ginseng root (Panax notoginseng)1000 mg (bonded to Phosphatidylcholine), Royal Jelly lyophylized (1.4% 10-hydroxydecenoic acid 50 mg, Cayenne fruit (Capsicum frutescens) 50 mg, Fo-ti root (Polygonum multiflorum) 50 mg, Yerba mate leaf (Ilex paraguariensis) 50 mg, Bee pollen 200 mg. Excipients: Di-Calcium phosphate, Microcrystalline cellulose, Cellulose gum, Vegetable stearic acid, Silica, Vegetable magnesium stearate and Vegetable resin.

Take 1 caplet with breakfast and 1 caplet with lunch, or as directed by your health professional.

60 caplets, blister packed.

Internal use. Non-irradiated.

Hypoallergenic caplet.

Visual.

Nu-Source® Natrarest®

Enhanced Valerian

⌂ **Nu-Life Nutrition Ltd.™**

Each caplet contains: Valerian root standardized extract 4:1 (Valeriana officinalis) 145 mg, St. John's wort standardized

7.5:1 (0.3% hypericin) (Hypericum perforatum) 100 mg, Catnip herb (Nepeta cataria) 50 mg, Passion flower herb (Passiflora incarnata) 50 mg, Hops strobiles (Humulus lupulus) 25 mg, Celery seed (Apium graveolens) 25 mg, Scullcap herb (Scutellaria lateriflora) 25 mg. Excipients: Di-Calcium phosphate, Microcrystalline cellulose, Cellulose gum, Vegetable stearic acid, Silica, Vegetable magnesium stearate and Vegetable resin.

Take 2 caplets at bedtime, or as directed by your health professional.

60 caplets, blister packed.

Internal use. Non-irradiated.

Hypoallergenic caplet.

Do not consume St. John's wort (Hypericum perforatum) during pregnancy.

Nu-Source® Tranquility®

Enhanced Standardized St. John's Wort

⌂ **Nu-Life Nutrition Ltd.™**

Each caplet contains: St. John's wort standardized 7.5:1 extract (0.3% hypericin) (Hypericum perforatum) 100 mg, Oat straw (Avena sativa) 75 mg, Lavender flowers (Lavendula officinalis 125 mg, Vervain herb (Verbena officinalis) 225 mg. Excipients: Di-Calcium phosphate, Microcrystalline cellulose, Cellulose gum, Vegetable stearic acid, Silica, Vegetable magnesium stearate and Vegetable resin.

Take 1 caplet with breakfast

and 1 caplet with dinner, or as directed by your health professional.

60 caplets, blister packed.

Internal use. Non-irradiated.

Hypoallergenic caplet.

Do not consume St. John's wort (Hypericum perforatum) during pregnancy.

Nu-Source® WearGuard

Enhanced Standardized Devil's Claw

⌂ **Nu-Life Nutrition Ltd.™**

Each caplet contains: Devil's claw secondary root standardized 5:1 extract (5% harpagosides) (Harpagophytum procumbens) 100 mg, Rheumatism root (Dioscorea villosa) 100 mg, Wintergreen leaf (Gaultheria procumbens) 25 mg, Tumeric rhizome standardized 30:1 extract (95% curcumin) (Curcuma longa) 50 mg. Excipients: Di-Calcium phosphate, Microcrystalline cellulose, Cellulose gum, Vegetable stearic acid, Silica, Vegetable magnesium stearate and Vegetable resin.

Take 1 caplet with each meal (3 daily), or as directed by your health professional.

60 caplets, blister packed.

Internal use. Non-irradiated.

Hypoallergenic caplet.

Do not consume Devil's claw (Harpagophytum procumbens) during pregnancy.

Nutribiotic Liquid Concentrate

⌂ **Nutribiotic**

⚱ Contains: Grapefruit seed extract.

▣ Available in 2 oz and 4 oz. Also available in tablet and capsule.

🔲 Internal and external use. Organic.

○ Liquid.

✋ Never use full strength, do not put in eyes.

Nutribiotic Skin Spray

⌂ **Nutribiotic**

⚱ Contains: Deionized water, Citricidal (GSE), Alcohol, Essential oils of Tea tree and Lemon.

✋ Spray 3-4 times daily on affected area.

▣ Available in 4 oz. spray bottle.

🔲 External use only.

○ Liquid.

Nutricap Capsules

⌂ **Yves Ponroy**

⚱ Contains: Walnut oil, soft gelatin capsule (gelatin, glycerol), Lithothamnium, Wheat germ extract, Coating agent:

Yellow beeswax, Emulsifier: Soya lecithin.

✋ Take 2 capsules daily for a minimum of 2 months.

▣ Available in 40 capsules per box in blister packs.

🔲 Internal use.

▭ Capsule.

Nux Vom.
Homeopathic Remedy

⌂ **A. Nelson & Company Ltd.**

⚱ Each pillule contains: Nux vomica 6c.

✋ Take 2 pillules every 2 hours for the first 6 doses, then 4 times daily for up to 5 days. Pillules should be sucked or chewed and taken between meals.

▣ 84 pillules/globules per bottle.

🔲 Internal use.

⊘ Pillule/globule.

Oak
Bach Flower Remedy

⌂ **Bach Flower Remedies® Ltd.**

⚱ Contains: Quercus robur 5x in 27% grape alcohol solution.

✋ Take 2 drops under the tongue 4 times daily or 2 drops in a small glass of spring water and sip at intervals.

▣ 10 ml with dropper.

🔲 Internal use.

○ Liquid.

Occhi Belli
with Eyebright and Bilberry

⌂ **Albi Imports Ltd.**

⚱ Each capsule contains: Eyebright 4:1 150 mg, Bilberry 5:1 100 mg, Grape seed extract 50 mg, Bioflavonoids extract 4:1 50 mg, Rutin 4:1 50 mg, Kelp 50 mg.

✋ Take 1 capsule 3 times daily.

▣ Available in 30, 60, 90 and 180 capsules.

▭ Capsule.

📷 Visual.

Ocean Formula
Glucosamine/Chondroitin Sulphate Complex

⌂ **Scandinavian Natural Health & Beauty Products**

⚱ Each capsule contains: Glucosamine sulphate 250 mg, Chondroitin sulphate 75 mg, Sea cucumber 50 mg, EPA 40 mg, DHA 100 mg (Omega-3 fatty acids), Shark liver oil 175 mg (containing alkylglycerols), Vitamin E 10 mg.

✋ Take 4 capsules daily for a body weight less than 150 lbs, 6 capsules daily for a body weight of 150-200 lbs, 8 capsules daily for a body weight of more than 200 lbs.

Available in 60 and 120 capsules

Internal use.

Capsule.

Ocu-Force™

Plus Lutein

Prairie Naturals®

Each capsule contains: Beta carotene (Provitamin A) 6,666 IU, Vitamin A (Palmitate) 1,000 IU, Vitamin B2 (Riboflavin) 15 mg, Pantothenic acid 10 mg, Vitamin B3 (Niacin) 10 mg, Folic acid .05 mg, Biotin 20 mcg, Vitamin C (Ascorbic acid) 150 mg, Vitamin E (d-alpha Tocopheryl succinate) 50 IU. Minerals: Calcium (HVP* chelate/citrate) 50 mg, Magnesium (HVP* chelate/citrate) 50 mg, Selenium (HVP* chelate/citrate) 20 mcg, Zinc (HVP* chelate/citrate) 5 mg. Lipotropic factors: Choline 25 mg, Inositol 25 mg, L-Methionine 25 mg. Non-medicinal ingredients: Lutein (100% natural from marigold flowers) 2 mg, Zeaxanthin (100% natural from marigold flowers) 88 mcg, Citrus bioflavonoids 50 mg, L-Glutamine 10 mg, Taurine 20 mg, Bilberry (Vaccinium myrtillus) 30 mg, Schisandra berries (Schisandra sinensis) 25 mg, in a whole food base containing carrot powder (organic) 10 mg, Spirulina (Blue-Green algae) 10 mg. *Hydrolyzed vegetable protein.

Take 1-3 capsules daily with meals or as directed by a physician.

Available in 180 capsules.

Internal use. Certified free of yeast, gluten, starch, soya, egg, dairy, artificial color or preservatives.

Capsule.

Visual.

Olbas Oil

Synpharma

Each 100 g contains: Oils of Eucalypt. glob. 36.5 g, Peppermint 34.7 g, Cajeput 25.0 g, Wintergreen 1.6 g, Cloves 0.2 g, Juniper 2.0 g.

Apply a few drops of Olbas oil and massage the skin, then cover with woolen material.

Available in 60 cc.

External use and inhalation.

Oil.

Caution: Discontinue use if irritation develops.

Olive

Bach Flower Remedy

Bach Flower Remedies® Ltd.

Contains: Olea europaea 5x in 27% grape alcohol solution.

Take 2 drops under the tongue 4 times daily or 2 drops in a small glass of spring water and sip at intervals.

10 ml with dropper.

Internal use.

Liquid.

Optibiol

Yves Ponroy

Contains: Fish flesh oil rich in eicosapentaenoic acid (EPA) and docosahexaenoic acid (DHA), Carrot oleoresin rich in natural Beta-carotene, Yeast rich in Chromium, Bilberries extract rich in anthocyanosids, yeast rich in Zinc, Technological additive: yellow beeswax; purified cerebral phospholipids on Silica, Emulsifier: Soya lecithin; Miscellaneous vegetable oils concentrate rich in natural vitamin E.

Take 2 capsules daily for a minimum of 2 months.

Available in 40 capsules per box in blister packs.

Internal use.

Capsule.

Orange

Essential Oil

Bach-Karooch Ltd.

Contains: Citrus sinensis 100%.

Two parts Essential oil must be diluted in 98 parts vegetable oil before applying to the skin. Consult Aromatherapy literature for specific methods of use and directions for each oil.

10 ml in amber bottle with child-resistant cap and one-drop insert.

Oil.

Caution: due to high concentration, all oils may be harmful if improperly used! External use only.

Original Silica™

Scandinavian Natural Health & Beauty Products, Inc.

Each tablet contains: 405 mg Horsetail plant extract, containing 2% Silicon dioxide. Excipients: Microcrystalline cellulose, Magnesium stearate, Colloidal silicon dioxide.

Take 2 tablets daily.

Available in blister packs of 60 and 180 tablets per box.

Internal use. Contains water-extracted Silica from organic non-medicated Springtime Horsetail plants.

Tablet.

Osteo Formula

Quest Vitamins

Each tablet contains: Calcium (HVP* chelate) 125 mg, Magnesium (HVP* chelate) 125 mg, Vitamin C (Ascorbic acid) 50 mg, Vitamin D3 50 IU, Silicon (HVP* chelate) 125 mcg. Non-medicinal ingredients: N-Acetyl glucosoamine 125 mg, Betaine HCl 25 mg. Croscarmellose sodium, Magnesium stearate (vegetable source), Microcrystalline cellulose, vegetable stearin. CellCote coating: Vegetable cellulose complex. *Hydrolyzed vegetable (rice) protein.

Take up to 6 tablets daily, in divided doses with meals, or as directed by a health professional.

Available in 90 and 180 tablets.

Internal use. Easy-to-swallow CellCote coated tablet. Contains no artificial preservatives, color, flavors or added sugar, starch, milk products, wheat or yeast.

Tablet.

Osteo-Force™

Prairie Naturals®

Each capsule contains: Vitamin B1 (Thiamine HCl) 2.5 mg, Vitamin B2 (Riboflavin) 2.5 mg, Vitamin B3 (Niacinamide) 5 mg, Vitamin B6 (Pyridoxine HCl) 5 mg, Pantothenic acid 2.5 mg, Folic acid .1 mg, Vitamin B12 2.5 mcg, Vitamin C 25 mg, Vitamin D3 50 IU. Minerals: Calcium (HVP* chelate/citrate) 150 mg, Manganese (HVP* chelate/citrate) 75 mg, Magnesium (HVP* chelate/citrate) 5 mg, Potassium (HVP* chelate/citrate) 25 mg, Silica 5 mg, (Equisetum arvense) Zinc (HVP* chelate/citrate) 5 mg. Non-medicinal ingredients: Glucosamine sulfate 30 mg, Betaine HCl 5 mg. In a Greenfood nutrient base consisting of organic Alfalfa, Spirulina blue-green algae, Barley grass, Norwegian kelp powder and Nettle leaves. *Hydrolyzed vegetable protein.

Take 4-6 capsules daily after meals or as directed by a health professional.

Available in 90 and 180 capsules.

Internal use. Free of yeast, gluten, starch, soya, egg, dairy, artificial colors, preservatives, solvents or alcohol.

Capsule.

Visual.

Osteoporex
Marine New Era Kit Advanced Formula

New Era® Natural Products Inc.

This kit contains: Marine Formula Ingredients: Sea algae (naturally sourced Calcium oxide and Magnesium from Rhodophycean species) zedoary (curcuma zedoary), Ginseng. Marine Formula Supplements: Shark liver oil and gelatin.

Take 2 capsules of Marine Formula daily with a meal and 1 capsule of Marine Formula Supplement.

Marine Formula Supplement 30 capsules and Marine Formula 60 capsules.

Internal use. Preservative-free.

Capsule.

P.B.E. Supreme
Proanthocyanidin Complex

Nutra Research International

Each capsule contains: Proanthocyanidin 50 mg from Grape seed and Pine bark extract, Citrus bioflavonoids 150 mg.

Take 1-2 capsules daily. 6-10 capsules daily for therapeutic use.

Available in 60 and 120 capsules.

Internal use. Standardized Proanthocyanidin.

Capsule.

P.M.S.
Homeopathic Complex

A. Nelson & Company Ltd.

Each tablet contains: Graphites 6c, Nat mur 6c, Sepia 6c, Pulsatilla 6c, Lycopodium 6c, Lachesis 6c, Nux vomica 6c.

Suck or chew 2 tablets every 2 hours for 6 doses (12 tablets), then 2 tablets 3 times daily until symptoms subside.

72 tablets in blister packs.

Internal use.

Tablet.

P-5-P Plus
Vitamin B6 Metabolite with Magnesium

Klaire Laboratories, Inc., USA & Europe

Each capsule contains: Magnesium (Glycinate) 100 mg. Pyridoxal-5-Phosphate 50 mg. Added ingredient: L-Leucine.

Take 1 capsule daily or as directed by a physician.

Available in 100 capsules.

Internal use.

Capsule.

Padma 28®

Padma

Each tablet contains: Saussuria 40 mg, Iceland moss 40 mg, Margosa 35 mg, Cardamon 30 mg, Myrobalan 30 mg, Red sandalwood 30 mg, Allspice 25 mg, Bengal quince 20 mg, Calcium sulphate 20 mg, Columbine 15 mg, Knot-grass 15 mg, Ribwort 15 mg, Licorice 15 mg, Golden cinquefoil 15 mg, Cloves 12 mg, Valerian 10 mg, Ginger-lily 10 mg, Heartlived sida 10 mg, Wild lettuce 6 mg, Marigold 5 mg, Camphor 4 mg.

Take 2 tablets 3 times daily for first week, 2 tablets thereafter.

Available in 120 tablets.

Internal use. Manufactured in Switzerland. Padma 28 is based on an ancient Tibetan recipe.

Tablet.

Visual.

Pagosid™ Devil's Claw Root 410

Dr. Dunner AG

Each tablet contains: 410 mg of standardized hydrous extract derived from 820 mg of Devil's claw secondary root.

Take 1 tablet with liquid 10 minutes before meals three times daily. A course of tablets should be taken for at least 20 weeks.

Available in 84 and 150 tablets blisterpacked.

Internal use.

Tablet.

Visual.

Pain Ease Formula

Natural Factors® Nutritional Products Ltd.

Each capsule contains: White willow bark extract (3.5% Salicin) (Salix alba) 100 mg, Valerian 4:1 extract (Valeriana officinalis) 25 mg, Black Cohosh 4:1 extract (Cimicifuga racemosa) 25 mg, White willow bark powder (Salix alba) 100 mg, Wood betony powder (Stachys officinalis) 100 mg, in a gelatin capsule with rice protein.

Take 1-3 capsules daily.

Available in 90 capsules.

Internal use. Contains no artificial preservatives, color, dairy, sweeteners, starch, wheat or yeast.

Capsule.

Do not consume Black Cohosh during pregnancy.

Visual.

PainAway®

Traditional Pain Remedy

Flora Manufacturing & Distributing Ltd.

Each capsule contains: Willow bark extract 500 mg, Willow bark powder 30 mg, containing 55 mg standardized salicin, in Vegicaps® (non-animal source, easily digested capsules).

Take 2 capsules as needed, up to 3 times daily (or as directed by a physician), preferably with food.

Available in amber bottle of 30 capsules.

Internal use.

Vegetarian capsule.

Unknown.

If you expect to undergo surgery, including dental surgery within 6 to 10 days of taking PainAway, consult your physician. Overdoses can occur. Consult a physician before taking this product under the following conditions: when taking other salicylates, if taking medicines for anticoagulation (thinning of the blood), diabetes or gout, during pregnancy (especially in the last trimester), or nursing, if pain, fever or inflammation persists, if allergic to salicylates, if taking any other non-steroidal anti-inflammatories (including other salicylates, if suffering from gastrointestinal bleeding, intestinal ulcers, or bleeding, if there is a history of asthma or other allergic conditions, if suffering from severe anemia. Since our product produces low salicylic acid levels, we recommend that PainAway not be used in the treatment of gout. This package contains enough drug to seriously harm a child. PainAway should not be used for prevention of heart disease, migraines or strokes because it presently has not been proven to inhibit platelet-activating factors. Children under 16 years should not use this product.

Visual.

Palmarosa

Essential Oil

Bach-Karooch Ltd.

Contains: Cymbopogen martinii 100%.

Two parts Essential oil must be diluted in 98 parts vegetable oil before applying to the skin. Consult Aromatherapy literature for specific methods of use and directions for each oil.

10 ml in amber bottle with child-resistant cap and one-drop insert.

Oil.

Caution: due to high concentration, all oils may be harmful if improperly used! External use only.

Panax Ginseng

Nature's Herbs®

Contains: EuroQuality® extract of Panax ginseng standardized for 20% ginsenosides, 6 g, in pure alpine spring water. Pure grain alcohol, 20% by volume.

Take 10–30 drops 3 times daily with water or juice. Shake well before use.

Available in 1 oz (30 ml).

Internal use.

Tincture.

Panax Ginseng C.A. Meyer

Standardized Extract

Natural Factors® Nutritional Products Ltd.

Each capsule contains: Ginseng (Panax) extract (standardized for a minimum 7% Ginsenosides from Panax Ginseng C.A. Meyer) 100 mg, in a base of certified organic flaxseed oil.

Take 1-3 capsules daily or as directed by a physician.

Available in 30, 60 and 90 capsules.

Internal use. Standardized at the preferred concentration of naturally balanced active constituents, including balanced ratios of the different Ginsenoside groups Rg 1/Rb 1 at 0.5%. This Ginseng is a concentration of 4-6 year main roots.

Softgel capsule.

Visual.

Pancreatin & Enzymes

🏠 **Natural Factors®
Nutritional Products Ltd.**

⚗️ Each tablet contains:
Pancreatin (1 mg = 52 USP
units) 300 mg, Pepsin 100 mg,
Lipolytic enzyme 50 mg, (1 mg
= 2 USP units). Non-medicinal ingredients: Bromelain 50
mg, Ox bile 50 mg and
Cellulose 5 mg.

✋ Take 1 tablet at mealtime.

📦 Available in 90 and 180
tablets.

🔠 Internal use. Contains no artificial preservatives, color,
dairy, sweeteners, starch,
wheat or yeast.

⊘ Tablet.

📷 Visual.

Parsley Leaf

🏠 **Nature's Herbs®**

⚗️ Each 455 mg capsule contains:
Premium Parsley leaf.

✋ Take 3 capsules 3 times daily
with a large glass of water.

📦 Available in 100 capsules.

🔠 Internal use. Preservative-free.

💊 Capsule.

Patchouli
Essential Oil

🏠 **Bach-Karooch Ltd.**

⚗️ Contains: Pogostemon
patchouli 100%.

✋ Two parts Essential oil must be
diluted in 98 parts vegetable
oil before applying to the skin.
Consult Aromatherapy literature for specific methods of use
and directions for each oil.

📦 10 ml in amber bottle with
child-resistant cap and one-
drop insert.

💧 Oil.

⚠️ Caution: due to high concentration, all oils may be harmful
if improperly used!
External use only.

Peace River Bee Pollen
500 mg

🏠 **Natural Factors®
Nutritional Products Ltd.**

⚗️ Each capsule contains: Bee
pollen 500 mg.

✋ Take 2 capsules daily.

📦 Available in 90 and 180 capsules.

🔠 Internal use. Enriching Bee
Factors® Pollen originates
from the pristine Peace River
Valley, Canada. Product has
not been fumigated or irradiat-
ed.

💊 Capsule.

📷 Visual.

Peace River Bee Pollen
750 mg

🏠 **Natural Factors®
Nutritional Products Ltd.**

⚗️ Each capsule contains: Bee
pollen 750 mg.

✋ Take 1-2 capsules daily.

📦 Available in 90 capsules.

🔠 Internal use. Enriching Bee
Factors® pollen originates
from the pristine Peace River
Valley, Canada. Product has
not been fumigated or irradiat-
ed. Contains no artificial
preservatives, color, dairy,
sweeteners, starch, wheat or
yeast.

💊 Capsule.

📷 Visual.

Pepper Black
Essential Oil

🏠 **Bach-Karooch Ltd.**

⚗️ Contains: Piper nigrum 100%.

✋ Two parts Essential oil must be
diluted in 98 parts vegetable
oil before applying to the skin.
Consult Aromatherapy literature for specific methods of use
and directions for each oil.

📦 10 ml in amber bottle with
child-resistant cap and one-
drop insert.

💧 Oil.

🧴 Possible skin irritant.

⚠️ Caution: due to high concentration, all oils may be harmful
if improperly used!
External use only.

Peppermint
Essential Oil

🏠 **Bach-Karooch Ltd.**

Contains: Mentha piperata 100%.

Two parts Essential oil must be diluted in 98 parts vegetable oil before applying to the skin. Consult Aromatherapy literature for specific methods of use and directions for each oil.

10 ml in amber bottle with child-resistant cap and one-drop insert.

Oil.

Possible skin irritant.

Caution: due to high concentration, all oils may be harmful if improperly used! External use only. Avoid during pregnancy and when taking homeopathic remedies.

Petitgrain
Essential Oil

Bach-Karooch Ltd.

Contains: Citrus aurantium 100%.

Two parts Essential oil must be diluted in 98 parts vegetable oil before applying to the skin. Consult Aromatherapy literature for specific methods of use and directions for each oil.

10 ml in amber bottle with child-resistant cap and one-drop insert.

Oil.

Caution: due to high concentration, all oils may be harmful if improperly used! External use only.

Phosphagen HP™ (U.S.)

EAS

Contains: Dextrose, Phosphagen (HPCE pure Creatine monohydrate), natural and artificial flavor, Beet powder (for color), Citric acid, Disodium phosphate, Monopotassium phosphate, artificial color.

Mix 1 scoop (43 g) with 200-250 ml of water or juice. Drink 4 servings daily for 5 days, then maintain at 1–2 servings daily.

Available in grape, fruit punch and lemon-lime flavor. Available in single servings (43 g), 900 g or 1.8 kg.

Internal use. Creatine is a guanidine-derived, phosphorylated compound.

Powder.

Possible cramping or diarrhea if over consumed (non-toxic).

Visual.

Phosphagen™ (U.S.)

EAS

Contains: HPCE Pure creatine monohydrate.

Take 1 tsp. (5 g) to 250 ml of water or juice 1–4 times daily.

Available in 100, 210, 325, 510 or 1000 g.

Internal use. Creatine is the guanidine-derived, phosphorylated.

Powder.

Possible cramping or diarrhea when over consumed (non-toxic).

Visual.

Phosphorus
Homeopathic Remedy

A. Nelson & Company Ltd.

Each pillule contains: Phosphorus 6c.

Take 2 pillules every 2 hours for the first 6 doses, then 4 times daily for up to 5 days. Pillules should be sucked or chewed and taken between meals.

84 pillules/globules per bottle.

Internal use.

Pillule/globule.

Phyto Estrogen-Power®
Premium Women's Formula

Nature's Herbs®

Each 4 capsules contains: Soy germ isoflavone concentrate (standardized for 1.5% isoflavones) 1400 mg, Kudzu root (Pueraria Iobata) extract (standardized for isoflavones) 100 mg, Certified potency Korean ginseng (Panax) extract (standardized for 7% ginsenosides) 100 mg, Certified potency Dong quai (Angelica sinensis) extract (standardized for 0.8-1.1% ligustilide) 100 mg, Mexican wild yam extract 100 mg,

Boron 3 mg, Natural Vitamin E 800 IU in a base of Chasteberry (Vitex agnus castus) powder and Arrowroot.

Take 4 capsules daily.

60 capsules.

Internal use. Preservative-free.

Capsule.

Pine

Bach Flower Remedy

Bach Flower Remedies® Ltd.

Contains: Pinus sylvestris 5x in 27% grape alcohol solution.

Take 2 drops under the tongue 4 times daily or 2 drops in a small glass of spring water and sip at intervals.

10 ml with dropper.

Internal use.

Liquid.

Platinum Ginkgo Alert

Health Way Products

Each capsule contains: Standardized potency Ginkgo biloba (24% flavonoids and 6% terpene) 20 mg, Korean ginseng 30 mg, Ginger root 30 mg, Peppermint leaves 30 mg, Ginkgo Biloba leaves 295 mg, Schizandra berries 30 mg, Rosemary herb 30 mg, Yerba mate leaves 30 mg.

Take 2 capsules 3 times daily.

Available in 60 capsules.

Internal use.

Capsule.

Consult your health professional if you are on medication, have a medical condition, are pregnant or nursing.

Visual.

Platinum Mega Garlic 8000

Health Way Products

Each 500 mg capsule contains: Standardized Garlic powder made from 100% pure fresh Garlic, Allicin 4200 mcg, Allin 9500 mcg, Sulphur 3400 mcg, Thiosufinate 4750 mcg, Gamma-glutamylcysteins 8400 mcg.

Take 2 capsules daily, or as directed by a health professional.

Available in 60 and 120 capsules.

Internal use. Disintegration time 45 minutes in the small intestine. No yeast, sodium, fillers, binders or lubricants. Enteric-coated.

Capsule.

Visual.

Platinum Osteo Plus Glucosamine

Health Way Products

Each capsule contains: Glucosamine sulfate 250 mg, Curcumin (standardized 95%) 65 mg, Licorice root (4:1) extract 65 mg, Cat's claw 30 mg, Devil's claw root 30 mg, Yucca root 30 mg, White willow bark 30 mg.

Take 1-2 capsules 3 times daily.

Available in 60 and 120 capsules.

Internal use.

Capsule.

Should not be used during pregnancy or nursing.

Visual.

Platinum Rheuma Arthrite

Health Way Products

Each capsule contains: Alfalfa leaf 125 mg, Licorice root extract (4:1) 125 mg, Curcumin (standardized 95%) 125 mg, Cat's claw bark 3% 30 mg, Devil's claw root 30 mg, Yucca root 30 mg, White willow bark 35 mg.

Take 1 or 2 capsules, 3 times daily.

Available in 60 capsules.

Internal use.

Capsule.

Should not be used during pregnancy or nursing.

Visual.

PNE

🏠 **Nutra Research International**

⚗️ Contains: Cherry plum, Clematis, Impatiens, Rock rose, Star of Bethlehem, Hypothalamus, Willow bark, Elm, Amethyst water, Emerald water, 20% Ethanol USP.

✋ Children: 4 drops
Take 8 drops under the tongue 2-3 times daily on an empty stomach.

📖 Available in 1 oz.

Ⓘ Internal use. Hypoallergenic.

💧 Sublingual drops.

Pollen Hayfever

🏠 **Nutra Research International**

⚗️ Contains: Minute dilutions of various plants, including Ragweed and Dandelion, Emerald water, 20% Ethanol USP.

✋ Take 8 drops under the tongue 2-3 times daily on an empty stomach. Children: 4 drops.

📖 Available in 1 oz.

Ⓘ Internal use. Hypoallergenic.

💧 Liquid sublingual.

Pollen Plus Energy

🏠 **Natural Factors® Nutritional Products Ltd.**

⚗️ Each capsule contains: Bee pollen (Peace River) 300 mg, Gotu kola (Centella asiatica) 50 mg, Siberian Ginseng extract (guaranteed minimum 0.4% eleuthrosides) 50 mg, Royal jelly (minimum 5% 10-HDA) 50 mg.

✋ Take 1-2 capsules daily.

📖 Available in 90 and 180 capsules.

Ⓘ Internal use. Contains no artificial preservatives, color, dairy, sweeteners, starch, wheat or yeast.

💊 Capsule.

📷 Visual.

Pollinosan®

A. Vogel
Homeopathic Remedy

🏠 **Bioforce AG**

⚗️ Contains: Ammi visnaga 1x, Aralia racemosa 2x, Cardiospermum halicacabum 2x, Galphimia glauca 3x, Larrea mexicana 2x, Luffa operculata 6x, Okoubaka aubrevillei 2x, Alcohol content 70%.

✋ Take 20 drops, 3 times daily 15 minutes before meals or 2 tablets under the tongue, 3 times daily, 15 minutes before meals.

📖 Available in 30 ml or 90 tablets.

Ⓘ Internal use. Best results are achieved when started 1-2 weeks before the onset of the allergy season and continued throughout the period.

💧 Liquid.

Potassium Citrate
99 mg

🏠 **Natural Factors® Nutritional Products Ltd.**

⚗️ Each tablet contains: elemental Potassium (citrate) 99 mg.

✋ Take 1-5 tablets daily or as directed by a physician.

📖 Available in 90 and 180 tablets.

Ⓘ Internal use. Contains no artificial preservatives, color, dairy, starch, wheat or yeast.

⊘ Tablet.

📷 Visual.

Power Ginseng GX 2500+

🏠 **Power Health Products Ltd.**

⚗️ Each capsule contains: 100 mg of Korean ginseng extract containing 30% ginsenosides.

✋ Take 1 capsule daily in the morning.

📖 Available in 30 and 60 capsules.

Ⓘ Internal use. Contains both groups of ginsenosides, RG1, and RB1 (stimulant and sedative). Only 4-6 year old roots used.

💊 Capsule.

📷 Visual.

PowerVites Energy Complex™

Multi-Vitamin

The Green Turtle Bay® Vitamin Co., Inc.

Each 2 caplets contains: Vitamins: A (as Beta carotene) 5,000 IU, C (as Niacorbate) 250 mg, D (as d-alpha) 300 IU, E 25 IU, B1 (as Thiamine) 12.5 mg, B2 (as Riboflavin) 12.5 mg, Niacin (as Niacinamide) 50 mg, B6 (as Pyridoxine) 25 mg, Folate (as Folic acid) 300 mcg, B12 (as Cyanocobalamin) 12.5 mcg, Biotin 50 mcg, Pantothenic acid 50 mg, PABA 12.5 mg, Inositol 12.5 mg, Choline bitartrate 25 mg. Minerals: Calcium 165 mg, Magnesium (as glycinate) 120 mg, Zinc (as monomethionine) 5 mg, Selenium (as methionate) 15 mcg, Copper (chelate) 0.5 mg, Manganese (chelate) 5 mg, Chromium (as picolinate) 50 mcg, Potassium 25 mg, Boron (as Calcium boro gluconate) 1 mg. Bioflavonoids: Citrus bioflavonoids 25 mg, Rutin 5 mg, Hesperidin (citrus) 5 mg. Other: Bee pollen 250 mg, Betaine HCL 10 mg. In a base of Chondroitin sulfate, odorless garlic and five active Acidophilus-Bulgaricus-Bifidus species.

Take 2 tablets daily at mealtime.

Available in bottles of 100 and 200 tablets.

Internal use.

Tablet.

Premenstrual Ease PMS Formula® Capsules

Traditional Yin-Yang Herbals

Flora Manufacturing & Distributing Ltd.

Each capsule contains: Powdered aqueous extracts of: Chai hu (Bupleuri radix), Dang gui (Angelicae sinensis, radix), Bai shao (paeoniae lactiflorae, radix), Fu ling (Poriae cocos, sclerotium), Bai zhu (Atractylodis macrocephalae, rhizoma), Gan cao (Glycyrrhizae uralensis, radix), Mu dan pi (Moutan radicis, cortex), Xiang fu (Cyperi rotundi, rhizoma), Chuan xiong (Ligustici chuanxiong, radix), Chen pi (Citri reticulatae, pericarpium), Gan jiang (Zingiberis officinalis, rhizoma), Bo he (Menthae haplocalycis, herba); spray dried on a corn starch carrier. 1:5 aqueous extract.

For severe symptoms: Take 3-4 capsules daily with liquid. Take the capsules for 5 days. Stop for 2 days. Repeat cycle throughout the month. For mild symptoms: Take 3 to 4 capsules daily with liquid. Take the capsules for 5 days, starting 14 days after the onset of menstruation.

Available in 90 capsules of 450 mg each, in an amber bottle.

Internal use. As presented by Dr. Malik Cotter (Diplomate of Oriental Medicine).

Vegetarian capsule.

Do not use when suffering from a cold, the flu or when digestion is disrupted. Pregnant women should consult a physician before taking this formula.

Premenstrual Ease PMS Formula® Tonic

Traditional Yin-Yang Herbals

Flora Manufacturing & Distributing Ltd.

Each 500 ml contains: Purified water aqueous extracts of: Chai hu (Bupleuri radix), Dang gui (Angelicae sinensis, radix), Bai shao (Paeoniae lactiflorae, radix), Fu ling (Poriae cocos, sclerotium), Bai zhu (Atractylodis macrocephalae, rhizoma), Gan cao (Glycyrrhizae uralensis, radix), Mu dan pi (Moutan radicis, cortex), Xiang fu (Cyperi rotundi, rhizoma), Chuan xiong (Ligustici chuanxiong, radix), Chen pi (Citri reticulatae, pericarpium), Gan jiang (Zingiberis officinalis, rhizoma), Bo he (Menthae haplocalycis, herba).

Shake the bottle well before use. For severe symptoms: Take 3 tbsp. two to three times daily. Dilute with warm water, if desired. Take the formula until bottle is finished. Stop for 2 days. Repeat cycle throughout the month. For mild symptoms: Take 3 tbsp. two to three times daily, starting 14 days after the onset of menstruation. Take formula until bottle is finished.

Available in 500 ml and 450 mg capsules.

Internal use. No preservatives added. To prevent contamination, do not drink directly from bottle. As presented by Dr. Malik Cotter (Diplomate of Oriental Medicine). Shelf life after opening is 14 days.

Capsule.

Tonic.

Do not use when suffering from a cold, the flu or when digestion is disrupted. Pregnant women should consult a physician before taking this formula.

Premium Chondroitin and Glucosamine Sulfate

Quest Vitamins

Each capsule contains: Chondroitin sulfate 200 mg, Glucosamine sulfate (sodium free) 300 mg, Magnesium stearate (vegetable source). Capsule shell: Gelatin, Water.

Take 2 to 4 capsules daily or as directed by a health professional.

Available in 90 Capsules.

Internal use. Contains no artificial preservatives, colors, flavors or added sugar, starch, milk products, wheat or yeast.

Capsule.

Primrose™

naka Sales Ltd.

Each capsule contains: Gamma-linolenic acid 50 mg, Cis-linoleic acid 360 mg (from 500 mg of Evening primrose oil) Vitamin E (d-alpha Tocopherol) 14.9 IU.

Take 3-6 capsules daily, or as directed by a professional.

Available in 90 capsules.

Cold pressed. Contains no artificial preservatives, colors, dairy, sweeteners, starch, wheat or yeast.

Gelatin capsule.

Pro-Men

With Saw Palmetto

naka Sales Ltd.

Each capsule contains: approx. 525 mg of the following herbs: Saw palmetto (extract), Small flowered willow (herb), Cranberry (extract), Stinging nettle (herb), Gravel root (root), Pumpkin seed (extract).

Take 1 capsule 3 times daily with each meal.

Available in 150 capsules.

Internal use.

Gelatin Capsule.

Probiata®

L. Acidophilus

Kyolic Ltd.

Each tablet contains: L. acidophilus in a vegetable starch complex. Provides one billion live cells prior to expiration.

Take 1 tablet for adults (1/2 tablet for children under four) with a meal, twice daily.

Available in 30 tablets.

The Traveler's Acidophilus™ Probiata® L. acidophilus is heat-resistant.

Tablet.

Progess Wild Yam Gel

8% Standardized Extract

Nutra Research International

Contains: Deionized water, Wild yam extract, Chamomile, Chaste berry, Arnica, Vitamin E, Carbomer (plant-based gum), Phenoxyethanol.

On a daily basis, alternate one of the following areas for application: under arms, breasts, inner thighs, under jaw.

Available in 2 oz.

External use.

Gel.

Not for use by pregnant or lactating women.

ProOptibol®

Performance Drink Mix

Next Nutrition

Contains: Pro Opticarb-AGI [branch-chain and straight-chain glucose polymers from corn hybrids and rice with xylitol], ProPeptone [a partially predigested blend of proteins from whey: B-Lactoglobulin, Lactalbumin, Lactoferrin, Immunoglobulin, with hydrolyzed eggwhite (a source of peptide-bonded and free-form amino acids) L-leucine, L-arginine, L-carnitine, Ornithine alpha-keto glutarate], F-Polyaminolactate (from pure crystalline D-fructose, Calcium lactate, L-arginine, L-glutamine, L-leucine, L-valine), Calcium caseinate, Potassium caseinate, VitaForte (bioactive vitamin-mineral mixture Potassium phosphate, Calcium carbonate, Magnesium oxide, Zinc gluconate, Potassium succinate, Vitamin E acetate, Ascorbic acid, Calcium pantothenate, Trimethylglycine, Molybdenum aspartate, Selenium aspartate, Manganese gluconate, Ferrous fumarate, Potassium iodide, Calcium glycerophosphate, Retinyl palmitate, Pyridoxine HCL, Niacin, Riboflavin, Thiamine, Pyridoxine alpha-ketoglutarate, Ferulic acid, Inosine, Folic acid, Biotin, Ergocalciferol, Cyanocobalamin, Carnosine, Lipoic acid, Pantetheine, Betacarotene, Ferrous succinate) Lecithin, Structured lipid complex (medium chain triglycerides with omega-3 fatty acids) Vanilla, Cellulose gum, Citric acid, Chromium arginate, Chromium picolinate.

Add 2 scoops to water, juice or non-fat milk, before or after exercise.

Available in 2.2 lb. (1000 g).

Internal use. Adapted from post-operative nutrition, scientifically formulated low sodium, low-fat, low lactose, partially-predigested complete food.

Powder.

Visual.

Propolis Throat Spray

 **Natural Factors®
Nutritional Products Ltd.**

Contains: Licorice root, Forsythia fruit, Slippery elm bark, Cloves, Propolis, Myrrh, Goldenseal root and Echinacea root in a base of approx. 20% grain alcohol, vegetable glycerin and black cherry flavor. Contains 12% standardized Bee Propolis.

Spray 2-3 times in mouth as needed for sore throat and gum pain, for lubricating dry mouth and throat and also as a breath freshener.

Available in 30 ml.

Internal use.

Spray.

Visual.

Propolis Tincture Extract 65%

 **Natural Factors®
Nutritional Products Ltd.**

Each ml (1 ml = 30 drops) contains: Pure Propolis extract 65% in a pure grain alcohol base.

Take 10-15 drops 2 times daily before mealtime, put directly in the mouth.

Available in 30 ml.

Internal use.

Tincture.

Visual.

ProstCare Prost-Action
Formula for Men

**Natural Factors®
Nutritional Products Ltd.**

Each capsule contains: Saw palmetto berry extract (serenoa repens) 80 mg, (standardized to contain 95% fatty acids and sterols), Pygeum Africanum (Africanus prunus) 20 mg (contains 14% total sterols), in a base of pumpkin seed oil and certified organic flaxseed oil.

Take 1-2 capsules twice daily or as directed by a physician.

Available in 60 and 90 softgel capsules.

Internal use. Contains no artificial preservatives or color, corn, dairy, gluten, soya, starch or yeast.

Softgel capsule.

Visual.

Prost Cleanse Formula
Formula for Men

**Natural Factors®
Nutritional Products Ltd.**

Each capsule contains: Juniper berry 4:1 extract (2% volatile oil) (Juniperus communis) 50 mg, Uva-Ursi extract (10 % arbutin) (Arctostaphylos Uva-Ursi) 50 mg, Parsley 4:1 extract (Carum petroselinum) 50 mg, Siberian ginseng extract (0.4% eleutherosides) (Eleutherococcus senticosus) 25 mg, Kelp 4:1 extract (Fucus vesiculosis) 25 mg, Flax meal powder (Linum usitatissimum) 75 mg, Cool Capsicum powder (Capsicum frutescens) 50 mg, Gravel root powder

(Eupatorium purpureum) 50 mg, in a gelatin capsule with rice protein.

Take 1-3 capsules daily or as directed by a physicians.

Available in 90 capsules.

Internal use. Contains no artificial preservatives, color, dairy, gluten, soya, starch, sweeteners or yeast.

Capsule.

Visual.

Prost LB-7

Albi Imports Ltd.

Each capsule contains: Saw palmetto berry extract (Serenoa repens) 200 mg, standardized to 25% fatty acids, Pygeum African extract 300 mg, (contains 2–4% total sterols) 30:1 (10 mg) Juniper berries extract powder 100 mg, (Juniperus communis) 2:1 (50 mg), Uva ursi extract powder 100 mg, (Arctostaphylos uvaursi) 2:1 (50 mg), Pumpkin seed extract powder (Cucurbita pepo) 4:1 (65 mg), Stigmata maydis (Cornsilk) 50 mg, Buchu leaves (Barosama crenulata) 25 mg.

Take 1–2 capsules daily.

Available in 30, 60, 90 and 180 capsules.

Internal use.

Capsule.

Visual.

Prosta Kit
One Month Program

Flora Manufacturing & Distributing Ltd.

Formula 1 PALMITOL® Each capsule contains: Saw palmetto liposterolic extract (85-95% concentration), Zinc citrate, Vitamin B6.
Formula 2 FLAX-OMEGA® Each capsule contains: Flax seed oil (freshly cold-pressed from certified organic seeds).
Formula 3 PRO-ESSENCE® Each capsule contains: Prickly ash bark, Juniper berry, Burdock root, Slippery elm bark, Bearberry leaves.

The three formulas in the ProstaKit® are designed to be taken together over a one month period.

Palmitol 30 capsules, Flax-O-Mega 120 capsules, and Pro-Essence 90 Vegicaps® capsules.

Internal use. Contains Palmitol, a high potency quality Saw palmetto extract. Completely safe and natural.

Capsule.

Prostasan®
A.Vogel
Herb Extract

Bioforce AG

Each ml contains: Saw palmetto fruit 0.935 ml, fresh Golden rod herb 0.03 ml, fresh Echinacea herb 0.02 ml, fresh wild Aspen bark and leaf 0.015 ml.

Take 15-20 drops 3 times daily in a small amount of water, 15

minutes before meals. Salivate before swallowing.

Available in 50 ml.

Internal use.

Tincture.

At the onset of a prostate condition, the symptoms may be quite subtle, for instance, difficult urination, natural dripping, frequent need to urinate and heavy pulling feeling in the lower abdomen. Consult a physician if any of these symptoms appear or persist.

Prostate

Nutra Research International

Contains: Gingko biloba, energetic imprints of: Pituitary, Prostate, Testrate, 20% Ethanol USP, Amethyst water.

Children: 4 drops
Take 8 drops under the tongue 2-3 times daily on an empty stomach.

Available in 1 oz.

Internal use. Hypoallergenic.

Liquid sublingual.

Prostatonin®

Pharmaton

Each capsule contains: Standardized Stinging nettle (Urtica dioica) extract UR102™ 300 mg, standardized Pygeum africanum extract PY102™ 25 mg. Non-medicinal: Rape seed oil, Soya lecithin, Vegetable stearin. Capsule shell: Gelatin, Glycerol, Sorbitol, natural color.

Take 1 capsule twice daily with liquid after meals.

Available in 30 and 60 capsules.

Internal use. Contains no artificial preservatives, colors, flavors or added sugar, starch, milk products, wheat or yeast.

Capsule.

Protec Acidophilus
Non-Dairy

Natural Factors® Nutritional Products Ltd.

Each capsule contains: 4 billion active cells of the following specially cultured strains of probiotics: L.rhamnosus 80% 3.20 billion, L. acidophilus 10% 0.40 billion, B. longum 5% 0.20 billion, B. bifidum 5% 0.20 billion. FOS (Fructooligosaccharides: naturally occurring complex fructose molecules derived from chicory root) 200 mg.

Take 3 capsules daily on an empty stomach or at bedtime.

Available in 60, 90 and 180 capsules.

Internal use. Contains no artificial preservatives, color, corn, dairy, soya, starch or yeast. At time of manufacture guaranteed minimum 4 billion active cells per capsule.

Enterocoated capsule.

Visual.

Psyllium Husk

Nature's Herbs®

Each 567 mg capsule contains: Premium Psyllium seed husk dietary fiber.

Take 3-4 capsules 3 times daily with a full 8 oz. glass of water before or after meals.

Available in 100 capsules.

Internal use. Preservative-free.

Capsule.

Psyllium Seed

Nature's Herbs®

Each capsule contains: Wild countryside® Psyllium seed dietary fiber 610 mg.

Take 3-4 capsules 3 times daily with a full 8 oz. glass of water before or after meals.

Available in 100 capsules.

Internal use. Preservative-free.

Capsule.

Pulsatilla
Homeopathic Remedy

A. Nelson & Company Ltd.

Each pillule contains: Pulsatilla 6c.

Take 2 pillules every 2 hours for the first 6 doses, then 4 times daily for up to 5 days. Pillules should be sucked or chewed and taken between meals.

84 pillules/globules per bottle.

Internal use.

Pillule/globule.

Pure E
All Natural 400 IU

Klaire Laboratories, Inc., USA & Europe

Each capsule contains: Vitamin E (d-alpha tocopherol) 400 IU, also contains at least 30% mixed Tocopherols which includes d-Beta, d-Delta and d-Gamma. Derived from Soya.

Take 1 or 2 capsules daily or as directed by a physician.

100 capsules.

Contains no protein or added oils.

Soft gelatin capsules.

Pycnogenol®
French Maritime Pine Bark Extract™

Natural Factors® Nutritional Products Ltd.

Each capsule contains: Pycnogenol® 25 mg (French maritime Pine bark extract), in a base of microcrystalline cellulose.

Take 2 capsules daily or as directed by a physician.

Available in 60 capsules.

Internal use. Contains no artificial preservatives, colors, dairy, soya, starch, wheat or yeast.

Capsule.

Visual.

Quercetin Bioflavonoid Complex

600 mg

Natural Factors® Nutritional Products Ltd.

Each 600 mg capsule contains: Quercetin (Bioflavonoid) 250 mg, Bioflavonoid complex (lemon, orange, grapefruit) 250 mg, Bromelain 50 mg, Rutin 50 mg. Encapsulated in a gelatin capsule with vegetable grade Magnesium stearate (used as a lubricant).

Take 1-3 capsules daily.

Available in 60 and 90 capsules.

Internal use.

Capsule.

Visual.

Quintessence® Garlic Plus FOS

Standardized

Pure-Gar®

Each tablet contains: 100% Pure-Gar® Garlic 500 mg, Nutraflora™, FOS 500 mg.

Take 2 tablets, 2 times daily with meals.

100 Tablets.

Internal use. 100% Vegetarian. No after-odor. Disintegration time: 45 minutes in the stomach. Yeast free.

Tablet.

Quintessence® Garlic Plus Ginkgo

Standardized

Pure-Gar®

Each capsule contains: 100% Pure-Gar® pure Garlic powder 460 mg, Ginkgo biloba dry extract (cont. 24% ginkgo flavonoid glycosides) 40 mg.

Take 1 capsule, 3 times daily with meals.

250 capsules.

Internal use. No after-odor.

Capsule.

Quintessence® Garlic Plus Ginseng

Standardized

Pure-Gar®

Each tablet contains: 100 % Pure-Gar® garlic powder 300 mg, 100% pure American Ginseng root powder from Wisconsin (Panax quinque-folius), (Root to Health™) 350 mg.

Take 1 caplet, 3 times daily with meals.

Internal use. No after-odor. 60 caplets.

Caplet.

Quintessence® Maximum Allicin Garlic

Standardized

Pure-Gar®

Each caplet contains: 100% Pure-Gar® Garlic 600 mg.

Take 1 caplet, 2 times a day with meals.

100 caplets.

Internal use. No after-odor.

Caplet.

Quintessence® Organic Garlic

Standardized

Pure-Gar®

Each capsule contains: 100% Pure-Gar® pure organic garlic 500 mg.

Take 2 capsules, 2 times daily with meals.

80 Vegicaps®.

Internal use. Organic. Contains no gelatin or other animal by-products, artificial preservatives, color, flavor, sugar, starch, soy, wheat, dairy or yeast. 100% vegetarian. No after-odor.

Vegicaps.

Quintessence® Pure Garlic
Standardized

Pure-Gar®

Each capsule contains: 100% Pure Gar® Garlic powder 500 mg.

Take 2 capsules, 2 times daily with meals.

Available in 100 and 250 capsules.

Internal use. No after-odor.

Capsule.

Real Aloe Vera Gel

The Real Aloe® Company, Inc.

Contains: Aloe vera gel with less than 1% preservatives: Potassium sorbate, Ascorbic acid, Sodium benzoate, Irish moss (thickener).

Take 2 oz. 4 times daily and/or use topically.

32 U.S. fl. oz.

Internal and external use. Organic.

Gel.

In case of adverse allergic reaction, discontinue use.

Real Aloe Vera Juice

The Real Aloe® Company, Inc.

Contains: Aloe vera juice with less than 1% preservatives: Potassium sorbate, Ascorbic acid, Sodium benzoate.

Take 2 oz. 4 times daily and/or use topically.

32 US fl. Oz.

Organic. Internal and external use.

Juice.

In case of adverse allergic reaction, discontinue use.

Real Aloe Vera Ointment

The Real Aloe® Company, Inc.

Contains: 68% Aloe vera juice, Safflower oil, Glyceryl monostearate se, Isopropyl palmitate, Hydrogenated vegetable oil, Propylene glycol, Stearic acid, Glyceryl stearate/Peg-100, Cetyl Alcohol, Cetearyl, alcohol, Poloysorbate-60, Dimethicone, Methylparaben, Propylparaben, Quarternium-15, Xanthan gum, Tocopheryl acetate (Vitamin E), Retinyl palminate (Vitamin A), Ergocaleiferol (Vitamin D).

Apply ointment to affected area for relief of skin irritations.

External use only. Unscented.

Ointment.

Red Beet Juice

W. Schoenenberger

Contains: Pure natural pressed herb and plant juice from organically grown Red beet plants.

Shake bottle well before use. Take 3 or 4 times daily before meals 1 tbsp. diluted in water, milk or tea, one part juice to six parts liquid. For children 1 tsp. instead of tbsp. Unopened bottle will keep indefinitely: opened, for 6 days.

Amber bottle of 5.5 fl. oz.

Internal use. Organically grown in nearly ideal conditions in the Black Forest & Swabian uplands, where the air is pure the plants are gathered at the moment when their production of valuable ingredients is at its peak. The juices are extracted by specially designed hydraulic presses that ensure maximum recovery of all essential elements, making certain that not more than 2-3 hours elapse between harvesting, pressing and bottling.

Cellular plant juice.

Red Chestnut
Bach Flower Remedy

Bach Flower Remedies® Ltd.

Contains: Aesculus carnea 5x in 27% grape alcohol solution.

Take 2 drops under the tongue 4 times daily or 2 drops in a small glass of spring water and sip at intervals.

10 ml with dropper.

Internal use.

Liquid.

Red Clover Blossoms

Nature's Herbs®

Each 350 mg capsule contains: Red clover blossoms, Gelatin.

Take 3 capsules 3 times daily with a large glass of water.

Available in 100 capsules.

Internal use.

Capsule.

Red Clover Combination

Nature's Herbs®

Each 455 mg capsule contains: Red clover blossoms, Burdock root, Licorice root, Barberry bark, Yellow dock root, Cascara sagrada bark, Sarsaparilla root, Prickly ash bark, Buckthorn bark and Norwegian kelp.

Take 2-3 capsules 3 times daily with a large glass of water.

Available in 100 capsules.

Internal use.

Capsule.

Do not use if you have or develop diarrhea, loose stools, or abdominal pain. Consult your physician if you have frequent diarrhea. If you are pregnant, nursing, taking medication or have a medical condition, consult your physician before using this product.

Red Raspberry Combination

Nature's Herbs®

Each capsule contains: Red raspberry leaves, False unicorn, Blessed thistle, Blue cohosh root, Pennyroyal, gelatin.

Take 2 capsules daily with meals.

Available in 100 capsules.

Internal use.

Capsule.

Do not take if you are pregnant except during last six weeks of pregnancy.

Red Raspberry Leaf

Nature's Herbs®

Each 384 mg capsule contains: Wild countryside® Red raspberry leaves.

Take 1-3 capsules 3 times daily with a large glass of water.

Available in 100 capsules.

Internal use. Preservative-free.

Capsule.

Reishi Mushroom

Nature's Herbs®

Each 606 mg capsule contains: Premium Reishi mushroom.

Take 3-6 capsules daily with a large glass of water.

100 capsules.

Internal use. Preservative-free.

Capsule.

Rescue Cream
Homeopathic Cream

Bach Flower Remedies® Ltd.

Contains: 5x dilution of Helianthemum nummalarium, Clematis vitalba, Impatiens glandulifera, Prunus cerasifera, Ornithogalum umbellatus, Malus pumila.

Apply cream to more than the affected area. Can generally be used as a salve.

27 g tube.

External use only.

Cream.

Visual.

Rescue Remedy
Bach Flower Remedy

Bach Flower Remedies® Ltd.

Contains: Helianthemum nummularium 5x, Clematis vitalba 5x, Impatiens glandulifera 5x, Prunus cerasifera 5x, Ornithogalum umbellatum 5x, in grape alcohol solution.

Take 4 drops under the tongue as required or 4 drops in a small glass of spring water and sip at intervals.

Available in 10 or 20 ml bottle with dropper.

Internal use.

Liquid.

Visual.

RespirActin™ ®

Sun Force International

Contains: Rosemary, Honey, Witch hazel, Fenugreek seed, Black seed, King Solomon seed, Ginseng powder, Damiana leaves, Marshmallow, Sage, Juniper berries, Chamomile flowers, Cloves, Cinnamon, Spearmint, Thyme.

Available in 8 oz. and 32 oz. bottles.

Safe for children. No ephedra, caffeine or alcohol.

Herbal tonic.

RHEUMATICA
Homeopathic Complex

A. Nelson & Company Ltd.

Each tablet contains: Rhus toxicodendron 6c.

Suck or chew 2 tablets every hour for 6 doses, then 2 tablets 3 times daily until symptoms subside. Childen: half the adult dose.

72 tablets in blister packs.

Internal use.

Tablet.

Rhus Tox.
Homeopathic Remedy

A. Nelson & Company Ltd.

Each pillule contains: Rhus toxicodendron 6c.

Take 2 pillules every 2 hours for the first 6 doses, then 4 times daily for up to 5 days. Pillules should be sucked or chewed and taken between meals.

84 pillules/globules per bottle.

Internal use.

Pillule/globule.

Rock Rose
Bach Flower Remedy

Bach Flower Remedies® Ltd.

Contains: Helianthemum nummularium 5x in 27% grape alcohol solution.

Take 2 drops under the tongue 4 times daily or 2 drops in a small glass of spring water and sip at intervals.

10 ml with dropper.

Internal use.

Liquid.

Rock Water
Bach Flower Remedy

Bach Flower Remedies® Ltd.

Contains: Aqua petra 5x in 27% grape alcohol solution.

Take 2 drops under the tongue 4 times daily or 2 drops in a small glass of spring water and sip at intervals.

10 ml with dropper.

Internal use.

Liquid.

Rosa Mosqueta® Oil
Rose Hip Seed Oil

Aubrey Organics®

Contains: Rosa Mosqueta® Rose hip (Rosa rubiginosa) seed oil.

Apply 2–3 times daily to affected area.

Available in 0.36 oz.

External use only.

Do not apply to open wounds or deep cuts.

Rose Absolute
Essential Oil

Bach-Karooch Ltd.

Contains: Rosa centifolia 100%.

Two parts Essential oil must be diluted in 98 parts vegetable oil before applying to the skin. Consult Aromatherapy literature for specific methods of use and directions for each oil.

10 ml in amber bottle with child-resistant cap and one-drop insert.

Oil.

Caution: due to high concentration, all oils may be harmful if improperly used! External use only.

Rose Otto
Essential Oil

Bach-Karooch Ltd.

Contains: Rosa damascena 100%.

Two parts Essential oil must be diluted in 98 parts vegetable oil before applying to the skin. Consult Aromatherapy literature for specific methods of use and directions for each oil.

10 ml in amber bottle with child-resistant cap and one-drop insert.

Oil.

Caution: due to high concentration, all oils may be harmful if improperly used! External use only.

Rosemary
Essential Oil

Bach-Karooch Ltd.

Contains: Rosemarinus officinalis 100%.

Two parts Essential oil must be diluted in 98 parts vegetable

oil before applying to the skin. Consult Aromatherapy literature for specific methods of use and directions for each oil.

10 ml in amber bottle with child-resistant cap and one-drop insert.

Oil.

Caution: due to high concentration, all oils may be harmful if improperly used! External use only. Avoid during pregnancy or if epileptic. Do not use if you have high blood pressure.

Rosewood
Essential Oil

Bach-Karooch Ltd.

Contains: Aniba rosaeodora 100%.

Two parts Essential oil must be diluted in 98 parts vegetable oil before applying to the skin. Consult Aromatherapy literature for specific methods of use and directions for each oil.

10 ml in amber bottle with child-resistant cap and one-drop insert.

Oil.

Caution: due to high concentration, all oils may be harmful if improperly used! External use only.

Royal Jelly 250 mg
Standardized Extract

Natural Factors®
Nutritional Products Ltd.

Each capsule contains: Royal jelly extract (5% 10-HDA potency, regular royal jelly is 1.5% 10-HDA potency) in a vegetable oil and lecithin base. Equals 1000 mg of Royal jelly.

Take 1 to 3 capsules 3 times daily.

Available in 60 and 90 softgel capsules.

Internal use. Contains no artificial preservatives, color, dairy, sweeteners, starch, wheat or yeast.

Softgel capsule.

Visual.

Royal Jelly 500 mg

Natural Factors®
Nutritional Products Ltd.

Each capsule contains: Royal jelly 500 mg in a vegetable oil and lecithin base. Encapsulated in a soft gelatin capsule.

Take 2-4 capsules 3 times daily.

Available in 60 and 90 capsules.

Internal use. Contains no artificial preservatives, color, dairy, sweeteners, starch, wheat or yeast.

Softgel capsule.

Visual.

Ruta Grav.

Homeopathic Remedy

🏠 **A. Nelson & Company Ltd.**

⚗️ Each pillule contains: Ruta graveolens 6c.

✋ Take 2 pillules every 2 hours for the first 6 doses, then 4 times daily for up to 5 days. Pillules should be sucked or chewed and taken between meals.

📦 84 pillules/globules per bottle.

🔲 Internal use.

⊘ Pillule/globule.

Rutin 250 mg

🏠 **Natural Factors® Nutritional Products Ltd.**

⚗️ Each capsule contains: Rutin 250 mg. Encapsulated in a gelatin capsule with rice protein and vegetable grade Magnesium stearate (used as a lubricant).

✋ Take 1-3 capsules daily.

📦 Available in 90 capsules.

🔲 Internal use. Contains no artificial preservatives, color, dairy, sweeteners, wheat or yeast.

▭ Capsule.

📷 Visual.

Rutivite®

🏠 **Power Health Products Ltd.**

⚗️ Each tablet contains: Green buckwheat powder 570 mg, Rutin 30 mg.

✋ Take 2 tablets daily after food.

📦 Available in 66 tablets.

🔲 Internal use. 100% pure Green buckwheat. Both the flowers and leaves are used.

⊘ Tablet.

Salix SST Saliva Tablets®

🏠 **Scandinavian Natural Health & Beauty Products, Inc.**

⚗️ Contains: Sorbitol, Malic acid, Sodium citrate, Dicalcium phosphate, Citric acid. Excipients: Polyethylene glycol, hydrogenated Cottonseed oil, Silicon dioxide, Carboxymethylcellulose.

✋ Allow 1 lozenge to slowly dissolve in mouth as needed, up to 1 lozenge per hour.

📦 Available in blister packs of 30 and 120 tablets.

🔲 Internal use. Fresh citrus flavoring.

⊘ Lozenge.

Salusan Herbal Nerve Tonic

🏠 **Salus-Haus**

⚗️ Each capful (20 ml) contains: 2.7 g fluid extracts 1:7 in 15 % v/v alcohol of: Medicinal ingredients: Passion flower 428 mg, Balm leaf 279 mg, Rosemary leaf 237 mg, Valerian root 88 mg, St. John's wort herb 81 mg, Hops 41 mg, Lupulin 10 mg. Non-medicinal ingredients: Hawthorn leaf & blossom 279 mg, Hawthorn fruit 257 mg, Mistletoe herb 171 mg, Lemongrass herb 171 mg, Wheatgerm 147 mg, Bishopweed seeds 126 mg, Barley germ 145 mg, Bitter orange 101 mg, Bearberry leaf 36 mg, Horsetail herb 36 mg, Lemon peel 36 mg. Sweetened with honey and natural fruit concentrates.

✋ Take 1-2 capfuls before bedtime.

📦 Available in bottles of 10 ml trial size, 250 and 500 ml.

🔲 Internal use.

🍶 Tonic.

⚠️ This product may cause drowsiness. Do not drive or engage in activities requiring alertness and avoid alcoholic beverages.

Salusan Herbal Rest

Alcohol free

🏠 **Salus-Haus**

⚗️ Each capful (20 ml) contains: 1.8 g fluid extracts 1:16 of: Medicinal ingredients: Passion flower 632 mg, Balm leaf 496 mg, Rosemary leaf 486 mg,

Valerian root 80 mg, St. John's wort herb 74 mg, Hops 38 mg, Lupulin 10 mg. Non-medicinal ingredients: Lemongrass 156 mg, Wheatgerm 134 mg, Barleygerm 132 mg, Bitter orange 92 mg, Lemon peel 34 mg, Bearberry leaf 34 mg. Sweetened with honey and natural fruit concentrates.

Take 1-2 capfuls before bedtime.

Available in bottles of 250 ml or 10 ml trial size.

Internal use.

Tonic.

This product may cause drowsiness. Do not drive or engage in activities requiring alertness and avoid alcoholic beverages.

Sambu® Elderberry Mini Cleanse and Deep Cleanse

Flora Manufacturing & Distributing Ltd.

Mini Cleanse contains: One bottle of Sambu® Elderberry concentrate 500 ml, Sambu® 10 Elderberry tablets 400 mg each, Ten Sambu® Birch-Juniper capsules 650 mg each, Twelve teabags Uratonic® tea 1.6 mg each and Floralax® II 60 mg.
Deep Cleanse contains: Three bottles of Sambu® Elderberry concentrate 500 ml, 40 Sambu® Wild Grown Elderberry tablets 400 mg each, 30 Sambu® Birch-Juniper extract capsules 650 mg each, 24 Uratonic tea bags 1.6 g each, Floralax® II 200 mg, Seven samples of Epresat®

Herbal Multivitamin liquid formula 10 ml each, 15 tea bags of Paradise tea 2.5 g each.

Follow instructions in kit.

Available in 3 day and 10 day kits.

Internal use.

Capsule.

Herbal Tea.

Powder.

Tablet.

Tonic.

Not recommended for pregnant or lactating women, the wheelchair-bound, or those sensitive to honey. Consult your health care practitioner before undergoing any dietary modification.

Visual.

Samson Hair Conditioner™

Scandinavian Natural Health & Beauty Products, Inc.

Contains: Pollen extract (standardized), Aloe vera concentrate, Tea tree oil, Zinc oxide, Biotin. Excipients: Ethanol, distilled water, Vitamin E, citrus fragrance.

Rub gently into the scalp twice daily for 3 weeks. Pause 1 week. Repeat this process 3 times for a total period of 16 weeks.

Available in 3.5 fl. oz.

External use only.

Gel.

Samson Protein Plus™

Scandinavian Natural Health & Beauty Products, Inc.

Each tablet contains: Marine proteins and mucopolysaccarides, Vitamin C, Horsetail plant extract, Yeast extract, Vitamin E, Calcium gluconate, Grape seed extract, Zinc gluconate, Coenzyme Q 10, Betacarotene, Vitamin A, Selenium, Biotin, Vitamin D.

As a complement to Samson Hair Conditioner take 1 tablet twice daily with meals for 3 weeks, pause 1 week. Repeat this process 3 times for a total of 16 weeks.

Available in blister packs of 180 tablets per box.

Internal use. For maximum benefit, use together with Samson Hair Conditioner and Samson Silica for a 4 month period.

Tablet.

Samson Silica™

Scandinavian Natural Health & Beauty Products, Inc.

Each tablet contains: 405 mg Horsetail plant extract, containing 2% Silicon dioxide. Excipients: Microcrystalline cellulose, Magnesium stearate, Colloidal silicon dioxide.

As a complement to Samson Hair Conditioner, take 1 tablet twice daily with meals for 3 weeks. Pause 1 week. Repeat the process 3 times for a total of 16 weeks.

Available in blister packs of 180 tablets per box.

Internal use.

Tablet.

Sandalwood

Essential Oil

Bach-Karooch Ltd.

Contains: Santalum album 100%.

Two parts Essential oil must be diluted in 98 parts vegetable oil before applying to the skin. Consult Aromatherapy literature for specific methods of use and directions for each oil.

10 ml in amber bottle with child-resistant cap and one-drop insert.

Oil.

Caution: due to high concentration, all oils may be harmful if improperly used! External use only.

Sarsaparilla Root

Nature's Herbs®

Each 455 mg capsule contains: Wild countryside® Sarsaparilla (smilax) root.

Take 2 capsules 2-3 times daily with a full glass of water.

Available in 100 capsules.

Internal use. Preservative-free.

Capsule.

Saw Palmetto Power®

80 mg

Nature's Herbs®

Each capsule contains: 80 mg certified potency Saw palmetto berry extract concentrated and standardized for a minimum of preferred 85-95% fatty acids and biologically active sterols.

Take 2 capsules 2 times daily with a large glass of water.

Available in 60 softgel capsules.

Internal use.

Softgel capsule.

Saw Palmetto Power®

160 mg

Nature's Herbs®

Each capsule contains: 160 mg certified potency Saw palmetto berry extract concentrated and standardized for a minimum of preferred 85-95% fatty acids and biologically active sterols, in a base of Pumpkin seed oil.

Take 1 capsule 2 times daily.

Available in 30 softgel capsules.

Internal use. Preservative-free.

Softgel capsule.

Scandinavian Soy Diet Program®

Scandinavian Natural Health & Beauty Products, Inc.

Contains: Dehydrated mung-bean sprouts, Oat bran, Vitamin C, Vitamin E, Vitamin B3, Beta carotene, Vitamin B12, Folic acid, Vitamin D3, Vitamin B6. Excipients: Sorbitol, Dicalcium phospate, Microcrystalline cellulose, Magnesium stearate.

Take 2 caplets with a full glass of water 3 times daily between meals every other week.

Available in blister packs of 84 caplets (sufficient for one month's program) and a support pack including a diet plan, menus, recipes, suggestions for easy-to-do exercise programs and more.

Internal use. For best results combine with a low-calorie diet and light exercise.

Caplet.

Scleranthus

Bach Flower Remedy

Bach Flower Remedies® Ltd.

Contains: Scleranthus annuus 5x in 27% grape alcohol solution.

Take 2 drops under the tongue 4 times daily or 2 drops in a small glass of spring water and sip at intervals.

10 ml with dropper.

Internal use.

Liquid.

Scullcap

Nature's Herbs®

Each 425 mg capsule contains: Scullcap herb, gelatin.

Take 2-3 capsules 3 times daily with a large glass of water.

Available in 100 capsules.

Internal use.

Capsule.

Selenium 200 mcg

Natural Factors® Nutritional Products Ltd.

Each tablet contains: elemental Selenium (yeast) 200 mcg.

Take 1 tablet daily or as directed by a physician.

Available in 60 and 90 tablets.

Internal use. Contains no artificial preservatives, color, dairy, sweeteners, starch or wheat.

Tablet.

Visual.

Selenium Blue Shampoo
Treatment Shampoo for Hair and Scalp Problems

Aubrey Organics®

Contains: Coconut oil, Protein (soya), organic Jojoba oil, Aloe vera, Water, Amino acids (Cystine, Glutamic acid, Glycine, Proline, Leucine, Threonine, Arginine, Valine, Alanine, Lysine, Aspartic acid, Isoleucine, Phenylalanine, Tyrosine), Vitamin F-complex (Essential fatty acids), Selenium, Panthenol (B5) and herbal extracts, (Allantoin, Camomile, Balsam, Nettle, Coltsfoot, Horsetail, Rosemary, Sage, Indigofera). Preserved naturally with Citrus seed extract and Vitamins A, C and E.

Shampoo daily for best results.

Available in 8 oz.

External use only. Vegan. No synthetic detergents, all natural organic vitamin-mineral shampoo.

Shampoo.

Seleno Met
Selenium Supplement

Klaire Laboratories, Inc., USA & Europe

Each capsule contains: Selenium (L-Selenomethionine) 200 mcg. Added ingredients: Cellulose and L-leucine.

Take 1 capsule daily or as directed by a physician.

Available in 100 capsules.

Internal use.

Capsule.

Senna Extract

Nature's Herbs®

Each capsule contains: Wild countryside® Senna extract 25 mg. Other ingredients: Natural herbs (Ginger, Fennel).

Adults and children 12 years of age and over: take 2 capsules once or twice daily. Children 6 to under 12 take 1 capsule once or twice daily. Children 2 to under 6 years of age, take contents of 1/2 capsule once or twice daily. Children under 2 years of age consult a doctor.

Available in 100 capsules.

Internal use. Preservative-free.

Capsule.

Do not use laxatives when abdominal pain, nausea, or vomiting are present, or for a period of longer than 1 week unless directed by a physician. If you have noticed a sudden change in bowel habits that persists over a period of 2 weeks, consult a doctor before using a laxative. Rectal bleeding or failure to have a bowel movement after use of a laxative may indicate a serious conditions. Discontinue use and consult a doctor. If you are pregnant or nursing, seek the advice of a health professional before using this or any medication.

Sepia

Homeopathic Remedy

🏠 **A. Nelson & Company Ltd.**

⚗️ Each pillule contains: Sepia 6c.

👉 Take 2 pillules every 2 hours for the first 6 doses, then 4 times daily for up to 5 days. Pillules should be sucked or chewed and taken between meals.

📇 84 pillules/globules per bottle.

📘 Internal use.

⊘ Pillule/globule.

Shiitake Mushroom

🏠 **Nature's Herbs®**

⚗️ Each 606 mg capsule contains: Premium Dried Shiitake Mushroom.

👉 Take 1-3 capsules 3 times daily with a large glass of water.

📇 100 capsules.

📘 Internal use. Preservative-free.

💊 Capsule.

Shiitake Power™

🏠 **Nature's Herbs®**

⚗️ Each capsule contains: 100 mg certified potency Shiitake mushroom extract concentrated and standardized for a minimum of preferred 3 mg. KS-2 polysaccharides, synergistically combined in a base of Shiitake mushroom powder.

👉 Take 2 capsules daily with a large glass of water.

📇 Available in 60 capsules.

📘 Internal use. Preservative-free.

💊 Capsule.

Siberian Ginseng

🏠 **Albi Imports Ltd.**

⚗️ Each capsule contains: 518 mg pure Siberian ginseng (Eleutherococcus senticosus). Each tablet contains: 600 mg of Siberian ginseng extract powder (Standardized extract 4:1) 150 mg, Eleutherococcus senticosus.

👉 Take 1–3 capsules or tablets daily, preferably before morning meal.

📇 Available in 100 tablets or 100 capsules.

📘 Internal use.

💊 Capsule.

⊘ Tablet.

Siberian Ginseng Power Herb®

🏠 **Nature's Herbs®**

⚗️ Each capsule contains: 100 mg. Certified potency Siberian ginseng extract concentrated and standardized for a minimum of eleutheroside B 400 mcg, and D 300 mcg in a synergistic base of Wild countryside® Siberian ginseng root.

👉 Take 2 capsules 2-3 times daily with water.

📇 Available in 50 capsules.

📘 Internal use. Preservative-free.

💊 Capsule.

Silica Power®

🏠 **Nature's Herbs®**

⚗️ Each capsule contains: Silicic acid 30 mg equivalent to 23 mg of organic Silica. It is derived exclusively from 300 mg certified potency Springtime Horsetail extract, concentrated and standardized for a minimum of preferred 10% Silicic acid, equivalent to 7.7% Silica, in a synergistic base of Wild countryside® Springtime Horsetail grass.

👉 Take 1 capsule 2 times daily.

📇 Available in 60 capsules.

📘 Internal use. Preservatives-free.

💊 Capsule.

Silicea

Homeopathic Remedy

A. Nelson & Company Ltd.

Each pillule contains: Silicea 6c.

Take 2 pillules every 2 hours for the first 6 doses, then 4 times daily for up to 5 days. Pillules should be sucked or chewed and taken between meals.

84 pillules/globules per bottle.

Internal use.

Pillule/globule.

Silicea Gel

Anton Huebner GmbH & CO KG

Contains: Purified water, Silicic acid anhydride.

Take 1 tbsp. daily, straight or diluted in water or juice.

Available in 7 or 17 fl. oz.

Internal and external use. Available in US available as Body essential SILICA gel. Silicea is a colloidal preparation of natural silica in which microscopic particles of silica are finely dispersed in water.

Gel.

Visual.

Silymarin Complex

Standardized 80% Milk Thistle Extract

Inno-Vite Inc.

Each capsule contains: Silymarin 150 mg from 80% standardized Milk thistle extract, Dandelion 100 mg, Alfalfa concentrate 100 mg, Black radish 100 mg, Beet root powder 100 mg.

Take 1 capsule 3 times daily before meals.

Available in 60 and 120 capsules.

Internal use. Silymarin Complex contains no soy, yeast, sugar, starch, wheat, corn, milk, eggs, color, flavors or preservatives.

Capsule.

Visual.

Sincera® BiPhasic Cream

Scandinavian Natural Health & Beauty Products, Inc.

Contains: Jojoba oil, Octyl methoxycinnamate (UV ray filter), Tocopheryl acetate, Panthenol, Propylene glycol, Bee's wax, Avocado oil, Dimethicone, Cetyl alcohol, Phytic acid, Fragrance (white ginger and natural ylang ylang extract) Retinol (water-soluble Vitamin A), Sincera protein complex, Polyglucose, Pine bark extract. Excipients: Water, Propylene glycol, Glyceryl stearate, Methylparaben, Propylparaben, Steapyrium chloride, Triethanolamine, Cholesterol.

Use A.M and P.M. after cleansing with Sincera Preparative Cleansing Oil. Apply over entire face, neck and throat.

Available in glass bottles of 1.75 oz.

External use only.

Cream.

Sincera®Preparative Cleansing Oil

Scandinavian Natural Health & Beauty Products, Inc.

Contains: Soybean oil, Tocopheryl acetate, Chamomile extract, Rosemary extract, Lavender extract, Pine bark extract. Excipients: Phenoxyethanol, Butylparaben, Propylparaben, BHT.

Cleanser-oil. Use A.M. and P.M. Gently massage the oil onto face and throat with circular motions. Remove with a wash cloth dampened with warm water.

Available in glass bottle of 4 fl. oz.

External use only. A gentle yet effective cleanser. Suitable for all skin types, even oily, acne prone skin. A unique cleanser that dissolves "bad" surface oils (lipid peroxides), make up and "built up" dirt without destroying the skin's natural protective lipid barrier.

Sincera® Tablets

Scandinavian Natural Health & Beauty Products, Inc.

Each tablet contains: Marine proteins and mucopolysaccarides, Vitamin C, Horsetail plant extract, Yeast extract, Vitamin E, Calcium gluconate, Grape seed extract, Zinc gluconate, Coenzyme Q 10, Betacarotene, Vitamin A, Selenium, Biotin, Vitamin D.

Take 2 tablets daily for 90 days, thereafter 1 tablet daily in the evening. For maximum effect use together with Sincera Preparative Cleansing Oil and Bi-Phasic Cream.

Available in blister packs of 60 and 180 tablets.

Internal use.

Tablet.

SINUS

Homeopathic Complex

A. Nelson & Company Ltd.

Each tablet contains: Hydrastis 6c, Kali bich. 6c, Pulsatilla 6c, Thuja 6c.

Suck or chew 2 tablets every hour for 6 doses (12 tablets), then 2 tablets 3 times daily until symptoms subside.

72 tablets in blister packs.

Internal use.

Tablet.

Sisu B-Stress with Ginseng

Sisu™ Enterprises Co. Inc.

Each capsule contains: Vitamin B-1 25 mg, B-2 25 mg, Niacin 20 mg, B-6 50 mg, Pantothenic acid 100 mg, Folic acid 0.2 mg, Biotin 75 mcg, Choline 100 mg, Inositol 50 mg, Siberian ginseng 5:1 (0.4% eleutherosides) 50 mg.

Take 1 capsule daily with food.

Available in 60 capsules.

Internal use.

Capsule.

Do not use in cases of hypertension. Not to be used in conjunction with the anti-parkinson's drug Levodopa or with the anti-convulsive drug Phenytoin. Not recommended during pregnancy and lactation.

Sisu Calcium Magnesium with Vitamin D

Sisu™ Enterprises Co. Inc.

Each capsule contains: Calcium (citrate) 100 mg, Magnesium (oxide) 100 mg, Vitamin D (Cholecalciferol) 100 IU.

Take 2-6 capsules daily.

Available in 100 or 200 capsules.

Internal use.

Capsule.

Do not use in cases of kidney disease or hyperparathyroidism. Should not be taken with the antibiotic Tetracycline (at the same time).

Sisu Card-Floe II

Sisu™ Enterprises Co. Inc.

Each tablet contains: Beta carotene 1,000 IU, Vitamin A (fish liver oil) 2,000 IU, Vitamin E (d-alpha Tocopherol) 60 IU, Vitamin C (ascorbic acid) 400 mg, Thiamine mononitrate 18 mg, Riboflavin 3 mg, Pyridoxine hydrochloride 15 mg, Vitamin B-12 16 mcg, Niacin 7 mg, Niacinamide 2 mg, Panthothenic acid 33 mg, (calcium pantothenate) Folic acid 0.06 mg, Biotin 5 mcg, Calcium (citrate) 40 mg, Magnesium (oxide) 42 mg, Potassium (chloride) 42 mg, Iodine (Potassium iodide) 0.03 mg, Manganese (gluconate) 0.8 mg, Zinc (gluconate) 2.5 mg, Selenium (HVP* chelate) 20 mcg, Chromium (HVP* chelate) 13 mcg. *Hydrolyzed vegetable protein. Lipotropic factors: Choline (bitartrate) 66 mg, Inositol 4 mg, di-methionine 16 mg. Non-medicinal ingredients: Para aminobenzoic acid 19 mg, Betaine hydrochloride 13 mg, Lemon bioflavonoids 10 mg, L-cysteine hydrochloride 66 mg, natural citrus flavor.

Take 3 tablets daily with meals or as recommended by a health practitioner.

Available in 150 and 300 tablets.

- Internal use. Contains no dairy, wheat, corn, gluten, yeast or preservatives.

- Tablet.

Sisu Co-Q10

- Sisu™ Enterprises Co. Inc.

- Each capsule contains: Co Q10 (Ubiquinone) 30 mg.

- Take 1 capsule daily with meal.

- Available in 100 capsules.

- Internal use.

- Capsule.

- May cause occasional mild stomach upset.

- Not recommended during pregnancy and lactation.

Sisu Echinacea Glycerite

- Sisu™ Enterprises Co. Inc.

- Contains: Echinacea (whole plant extract) 1:1 1 g. In a base of Kosher vegetable glycerin, Grapefruit seed extract, natural flavors.

- Take 15-30 drops 3 times daily, between meals.

- Available in 30 ml raspberry, mint, orange, and tangerine flavors.

- Internal use. Organic.

- Tincture.

- Not recommended during pregnancy and lactation. Do not use in cases of auto-immune disorders (rheumatoid arthritis, AIDS, multiple sclerosis).

Sisu Enzymes Plus
Concentrated digestive plant enzymes

- Sisu™ Enterprises Co. Inc.

- Each capsule contains: Protease 12,000 HUT, Amylase 4,800 DU, Lactase 300 LacU, Lipase 48 LU, Sucrase 0.1 IAU, Cellulase 40 CU.

- Take 1-3 capsules with each meal.

- Available in 60 capsules.

- Internal use. Concentrated digestive plant enzymes.

- Capsule.

- Do not use in cases of known sensitivity to Aspergillus, acute pancreatitis, gastric and duodenal ulcers. Not recommended during pregnancy and lactation.

Sisu Ester ACES™

- Sisu™ Enterprises Co. Inc.

- Each capsule contains: Vitamin C (Ester C®Calcium ascorbate) 250 mg, Beta carotene 10,000 IU, Vitamin E (d-alpha Tocopherol) 200 IU, Selenium (selenite) 50 mcg.

- Take 1-2 capsules daily with meals.

- Available in 60 and 120 capsules.

- Internal use.

- Capsule.

Sisu Ester C

- Sisu™ Enterprises Co. Inc.

- Each capsule contains: Vitamin C (from Ester-C® Calcium ascorbate) 600 mg, Calcium (from Ester-C® Calcium ascorbate) 80 mg, Bioflavonoids (citrus) 100 mg.

- Take 1-3 capsules daily.

- Available in 60 and 120 capsules.

- Internal use.

- Capsule.

- May cause diarrhea in large doses and false positive test for urinary glucose

- Do not use in cases of hemosiderosis, hemochromatosis.

Sisu Ester C® Supreme

- Sisu™ Enterprises Co. Inc.

- Each capsule contains: Vitamin C (from Ester-C® Calcium ascorbate) 600 mg, Calcium (from Ester-C® Calcium ascorbate) 80 mg, Polysaccharides 100 mg,

Quercetin 50 mg, multi-antho-cyanidins (mixed berries) 50 mg.

Take 1-3 capsules daily.

Available in 60 and 120 capsules.

Internal use.

Capsule.

May cause diarrhea in large doses and false positive test for urinary glucose.

Do not use in cases of hemosiderosis, hemochromatosis, G6 PD deficiency.

Sisu EVC® Liquid

Sisu™ Enterprises Co. Inc.

Each 5 ml contains: Vitamin A (Palmitate) 1,000 IU, Beta carotene 1,000 IU, Vitamin C 100 mg, Zinc (glucomate) 2 mg, Vitamin B-6 (Pyridoxine HCl) 2 mg, Echinacea angusti-folia 1:2.5 100 mg.

Take 10 ml 3 times daily, with food.

Available in 120 ml grape, cherry and peach flavor.

Internal use.

Syrup.

Oral zinc can cause nausea.

Not recommended for infants or during pregnancy and lactation. Do not use in cases of auto-immune disorders (rheumatoid arthritis; AIDS,

multiple sclerosis), hemosiderosis and hemochromatosis. Should not be used in conjunction with alcohol or if you are taking Isotretinoin, Tetracycline, Levodopa, or Phenytoin.

Sisu EVC® Tablets

Sisu™ Enterprises Co. Inc.

Each tablet contains: Vitamin A (Palmitate) 10,000 IU, Vitamin C (Ascorbic acid) 500 mg, Vitamin B-6 (Pyridoxine hydrochloride) 20 mg, Zinc (gluconate) 15 mg, Echinacea extract (Angustifolia, Pallida, Purpurea) 1:1 300 mg, Bioflavonoids (citrus) 5 mg.

Take 2 tablets 3-4 times daily for 3-4 days. Take with food.

Available in 50 and 100 tablets.

Internal use.

Tablet.

Zinc may cause nausea if taken on an empty stomach.

Do not use in cases of hemochromatosis, hemosidero-sis or auto immune disorders (rheumatoid arthriti, AIDS, multiple sclerosis). Should not be used in conjunction with alcohol or if you are taking these drugs: Isotretinoin, Tetracycline, Levodopa, Phenytoin. Not recommended during pregnancy and lacta-tion or for infants.

Sisu Fos-A-Dophilus™

Sisu™ Enterprises Co. Inc.

Each capsule contains: Fructooligosaccharides (FOS) 200 mg, from inulin (chicory root), Lactic acid bacteria 4 billion organisms (L. aci-dophilus, L. rhamnosus, B. longum, B. infantis, B. bifidum, B. breve).

Take 3-4 capsules daily with meals.

Available in 90 capsules.

Internal use. Non-dairy.

Capsule.

Sisu Ginkgo Biloba Phytosome®

Sisu™ Enterprises Co. Inc.

Each capsule contains: Ginkgo biloba 50:1 extract Phytosome® 60 mg. Contains 24% flavone glycosides and 6% terpene lactones.

Take 1 capsule 3 times daily.

Available in 60, 120 and 360 capsules.

Internal use.

Capsule.

Mild stomach upset; possible headache during the first 1-2 days of use.

Sisu Glucosamine Sulfate Plus

With Shark Cartilage

🏠 **Sisu™ Enterprises Co. Inc.**

⚗️ Each capsule contains: Glucosamine sulfate 500 mg, Shark cartilage 250 mg.

👐 Take 3 capsules daily.

📦 Available in 120 capsules.

Ⅱ Internal use.

💊 Capsule.

Sisu Herbals for Skin: Acne

🏠 **Sisu™ Enterprises Co. Inc.**

⚗️ Contains: Dog rose, Glycerine mono-stearate, Cetyl alcohol, Aqua purificata, Borage seed oil, (26% G.L.A.), Primrose oil, Bioflavonoids, Vitamin E, Vitamin A, Calendula officinalis.

👐 Apply sparingly 3-5 times daily.

📦 Available in 30 g.

Ⅱ External use only. Not tested on animals.

🧴 Cream.

Sisu Herbals for Skin: Dermatitis

🏠 **Sisu™ Enterprises Co. Inc.**

⚗️ Contains: Manuka, Glycerine mono-stearate, Cetyl alcohol, Aqua purificata, Borage seed oil (26% G.L.A.), Primrose oil, Bioflavonoids, Vitamin E, Vitamin A, Calendula officinalis.

👐 Apply sparingly 3-5 times daily.

📦 Available in 30 g.

Ⅱ External use only. Not tested on animals.

🧴 Cream.

Sisu Herbals for Skin: Eczema

🏠 **Sisu™ Enterprises Co. Inc.**

⚗️ Contains: Fumatory, Glycerine mono-stearate, Cetyl alcohol, Aqua purificata, Borage seed oil (26% gamma linoleic acid), Primrose oil, Bioflavonoids, Vitamin E, Vitamin A, Calendula officinalis.

👐 Apply sparingly 3-5 times daily.

📦 Available in 30 g.

Ⅱ Not tested on animals.

🧴 Cream.

👶 Unknown.

🤚 External use only.

Sisu Herbals for Skin: Psoriasis

🏠 **Sisu™ Enterprises Co. Inc.**

⚗️ Contains: Pansy, Glycerine mono-stearate, Cetyl alcohol, Aqua purificata, Borage seed oil (26% G.L.A.), Primrose oil, Bioflavonoids, Vitamin E, Vitamin A, Calendula officinalis.

👐 Apply sparingly 3-5 times daily.

📦 Available in 30 g.

Ⅱ External use only. Not tested on animals.

🧴 Cream.

Sisu Leucoselect™

Grape Seed Phytosome®

🏠 **Sisu™ Enterprises Co. Inc.**

⚗️ Each capsule contains: Grape seed 100:1 extract Phytosome® 100 mg (standardized to contain 85-95% Proanthocyanidins bound to phosphatidylcholine (a fatty acid from lecithin) using the patented Phytosome® process).

👐 Take 1-3 capsules daily.

📦 Available in 60 Capsules.

Ⅱ Internal use. Contains no dairy, wheat, corn, gluten, yeast or preservatives.

💊 Capsule.

👶 Unknown.

Do not use in cases of known sensitivity to grape seed.

Sisu Liquid Cal-Mag with Vitamin D

 Sisu™ Enterprises Co. Inc.

Each 30 ml contains: Calcium (carbonate) 480 mg, Magnesium (oxide) 360 mg, Vitamin D (ergocalciferol) 200 IU. Herbal base: Prickly ash, Ginger, Fennel, Alfalfa.

Take 2 tbsp. daily.

Available in 340 ml mint, vanilla and strawberry flavor.

Internal use. No added sugar.

Liquid.

Do not use in cases of kidney disease or hyperparathyroidism. Should not be taken with antibiotic Tetracycline (at the same time).

Sisu Liv Select

Sisu™ Enterprises Co. Inc.

Contains: Indian ayurvedic herbs.

Take 6-9 capsules daily. Divide dose with meals.

Available in 100 capsules.

Internal use.

Capsule.

May cause soft stool.

Not recommended during pregnancy and lactation or for infants.

Sisu Mag-Citrate

Sisu™ Enterprises Co. Inc.

Each capsule contains: Magnesium (citrate) 100 mg, Malic acid 350 mg.

Take 1 capsule daily with food.

Available in 100 capsules.

Internal use.

Capsule.

May cause diarrhea in large doses.

Do not use in cases of kidney disease/failure, cancer. Should not be taken together (at the same time) with the antibiotic Tetracycline.

Sisu Milk Thistle Phytosome® Complex

Sisu™ Enterprises Co. Inc.

Each capsule contains: Milk thistle 30:1 Phytosome® 100 mg, (contains 15-20% silymarin), Globe artichoke leaf 4:1 50 mg, (contains 2% cynarin), Turmeric root 5:1 50 mg (7-9%cCurcumin), Dandelion root 4:1 50 mg.

Take 1 capsule 3 times daily.

Available in 60 and 120 capsules.

Internal use.

Capsule.

May cause loose stool and diarrhea.

Do not use in cases of cholelithiasis (gallstones), cholecystitis, intestinal obstruction. Not recommended during pregnancy and lactation.

Sisu Pycnogenol®

Sisu™ Enterprises Co. Inc.

Each tablet contains: Pine bark extract 25 mg. Guaranteed potency 85% proanthocyanadins.

Take 2-6 tablets daily.

Available in 30, 60, 90 and 180 tablets.

Internal use. Canada's first pine bark extract, from the maritime pine in France.

Tablet.

Unknown.

Sisu Select Echinacea Plus

Sisu™ Enterprises Co. Inc.

Each capsule contains: Echinacea angustifolia root 4:1 125 mg (4% echinacosides), Echinacea purpurea 20:1 125 mg (fresh juice extract).

Take 1 capsule 3-6 times daily.

Available in 60 capsules.

Internal use.

Capsule.

Not recommended for infants or during pregnancy and lactation. Do not use in cases of auto-immune disorders (AIDS, rheumatoid arthritis, multiple sclerosis).

Sisu Select Garlic

Sisu™ Enterprises Co. Inc.

Each caplet contains: Garlic 3:1 extract 250 mg (standardized to contain 2,500 mcg allicin and 5,500 mcg alliin).

Take 1-2 caplets daily with a meal. Do not chew.

Available in 60 caplets.

Internal use. No after-odor, enteric coated to be properly absorbed in the lower intestine. Contains no dairy, wheat, corn, gluten, yeast or preservatives.

Caplet.

Unknown.

Do not use in cases of known sensitivity to garlic. Should not be taken with the anticoagulant Warfarin.

Sisu Select PhytoVision

Sisu™ Enterprises Co. Inc.

Each capsule contains: Bilberry 100:1 (25% anthocyanidins) 25 mg, Grape seed 100:1 Phytosome® (15-20% proanthocyanidins) 25 mg, Ginkgo biloba 50:1 Phytosome® (24% glycosides, 6% terpene lactones) 30 mg, Multi-anthocyanidins (5% anthocyanidins) 25 mg, Lutein beadlets (5% pure lutein) 40 mg.

Take 1 capsules 2-4 times daily.

Available in 60 and 90 capsules.

Internal use.

Capsule.

Unknown.

Sisu Select Saw Palmetto Complex

Sisu™ Enterprises Co. Inc.

Each capsule contains: Serenoa repens (Saw palmetto fruit 4:1) 125 mg standardized to contain 25% fatty acids, Urtica dioica (Stinging nettle root 10:1) 75 mg, Curcubita pepo (Pumpkin seed 5:1) 50 mg standardized to contain 25% fatty acids, Pygeum africanum bark (30:1) 25 mg, Uva ursi (Bearberry leaf 4:1) 15 mg standardized to contain 10% arbutin.

Take 1 capsule 3 times daily.

Available in 60 and 120 capsules.

Internal use. Contains no dairy, wheat, corn, soya, gluten, yeast or preservatives.

Capsule.

Unknown.

Not recommended during pregnancy and lactation.

Sisu Select St. John's Wort

 Sisu™ Enterprises Co. Inc.

Each capsule contains: St. John's wort 5:1 300 mg; minimum 0.3% hypericines.

Take 1 capsule 3 times daily with meals.

Available in 90 and 180 capsules.

Internal use.

Capsule.

May cause photosensitivity; occasional stomach upset.

Not recommended during pregnancy and lactation. Should not be used in conjunction with anti-depressant medications, alcohol, or while operating heavy machinery; may cause drowsiness.

Sisu Supreme O-Live

Sisu™ Enterprises Co. Inc.

Each capsule contains: Olive plant extract (Olea europa) 5:1 500 mg, standardized to contain 4-6% oleuropein.

Take 1 capsule 1-4 times daily, between meals.

Available in 90 capsules.

Internal use.

Capsule.

Unknown.

Sisu Woman Changes

Sisu™ Enterprises Co. Inc.

Each capsule contains: Black cohosh 4:1 (1% terpene glycosides) 150 mg, Soy bean complex (with isoflavone glycosides, genistein and daidzin) 50 mg, Dong quai 4:1 (1% ligustilide) 150 mg, Wild yam 4:1 (10% disgenine) 50 mg, St. John's wort 4:1 (0.3% hypericin) 200 mg.

Take 1 capsule 2-3 times daily.

Available in 60 capsules.

Internal use.

Capsule.

May cause nausea, dizziness.

Not recommended during pregnancy and lactation. Do not take in conjunction with any anti-depressant or hormone replacement.

Sisu Woman Maxi-Cal

Sisu™ Enterprises Co. Inc.

Each tablet contains: Calcium (citrate) 275 mg, Magnesium (citrate) 137.5 mg, Vitamin D (Ergocalciferol) 100 IU.

Take 1 tablet 3 times daily with meals.

Available in 100 tablets.

Internal use.

Tablet.

Do not use in cases of kidney disease or hyperparathyroidism. Should not be used at the same time as the antibiotic Tetracycline.

Sisu Woman PMS

Sisu™ Enterprises Co. Inc.

Each capsule contains: Chaste tree 5:1 (0.75% aucubin) 100 mg, Dandelion root 4:1 (25% inulin) 200 mg, St. John's wort 3:1 (0.3% hypericin) 225 mg.

Take 1-3 capsules daily.

Available in 90 capsules.

Internal use. Standardized herbal formula.

Capsule.

May cause mild gastro-intestinal upset, mild rash with itching.

Not recommened during pregnancy and lactation, or for infants and children; Do not take in conjunction with anti-depressant medication or prescription hormone replacement therapy.

SKINVITAL®
Herbal Blend of Oily Extracts

Inno-Vite Inc.

Contains: all-natural oily extracts from: Soya hispida, Helianthus, Rape, Foeniculum vulgare, Pinpinela anisum, Peppermint.

1 tbsp. taken 2-6 times daily.

Available in 500 ml.

Internal use. SKINVITAL® is absorbed by osmosis through the mucous membranes of the mouth. Does not contain sugar, mineral oil, animal products, artificial colors, flavors or preservatives.

Liquid.

Those allergic to Sesame, Sunflower, Canola or Soya should not consume this product.

Visual.

SKINVITAL® Cream

Inno-Vite Inc.

Contains: Purified water, Castor oil, Triglycerides, Poly-Acrylamide, Isoparaffin, Laureth 7, Hydroxypropyl Methyl-Cellulose, Bovine cartilage, Citric acid, Glucose oxidase, Lactoperoxidase, Glucose.

Apply twice daily over cleansed skin.

Available in 60 g.

External use. Odorless and natural with no chemical preservatives.

Cream.

Visual.

Sleep Relax Formula

**Natural Factors®
Nutritional Products Ltd.**

Each capsule contains:
Valerian 4:1 extract (2% volatile oil) (Valeriana officinalis) 100 mg, Passion flower 4:1 extract (Passiflora incarnata) 50 mg, Hops 5:1 extract (Humulus lupulus) 25 mg, Skullcap powder (Scutellaria laterifolia) 100 mg, Hops powder (Humulus lupulus) 50 mg, in a gelatin capsule with rice protein.

Take 1-3 capsules daily.

Available in 90 capsules.

Internal use. Contains no artificial preservatives, color, dairy, sweeteners, starch, wheat or yeast.

Capsule.

Visual.

Slippery Elm Inner Bark

Nature's Herbs®

Each capsule contains: Wild countryside® Slippery elm inner bark 340 mg.

For oral health, adults and children 2 years of age and older: open 2 capsules and allow contents to dissolve slowly in the mouth, or prepare as a tea with honey. May be repeated every hour for as long as needed or as directed by a dentist or doctor. Children under 2 years of age consult a dentist or doctor. For stomach irritations, adults take 2-3 capsules as often as needed.

Available in 100 capsules.

Internal use. Preservative-free.

Capsule.

If sore throat is severe, persists for more than 2 days, is accompanied or followed by fever, headache, rash, nausea, or vomiting, consult a doctor promptly. If sore mouth symptoms do not improve in 7 days, see your dentist or doctor promptly. If stomach symptoms persist, stop this medication and consult your physician. If you are pregnant or nursing, seek the advice of a health professional before using this or any medication.

Spikenard

Essential Oil

Bach-Karooch Ltd.

Contains: Nardostachys jatamansi 100%.

Two parts Essential oil must be diluted in 98 parts vegetable oil before applying to the skin. Consult Aromatherapy literature for specific methods of use and directions for each oil.

10 ml in amber bottle with child-resistant cap and one-drop insert.

Oil.

Caution: due to high concentration, all oils may be harmful if improperly used!
External use only.

Spirulina Pacifica™

Nutrex® Inc.

Each tablet contains: certified organic Spirulina 500 mg, Silica 4 mg.
Powder contains: certified organic Spirulina.

Take 6-15 tablets daily or 1 or more tsp. daily. Powder-mix in juice, fruit smoothies or sprinkle on food.

Available in 100, 200 and 400 cold pressed tablets or 5 oz. and 16 oz. powder.

Internal use. Organic. Pesticide-free, non-irradiated. Packed in glass to prevent oxidation of key nutrients.

Powder.

Tablet.

Spirulina Pacifica™

Crystal Flakes

Nutrex® Inc.

Contains: Spirulina (95%), Soy lecithin (5%).

Sprinkle on foods such as rice, pasta, salads, soups & dips, or add 2 or more tsp. to a fruit smoothie for a tasty and nutritious boost.

Available in 0.75 oz. and 7 oz. bottle.

Internal use. Certified organic. Pesticide free, non-irradiated. Provides 30 mg of Gamma linolenic acid per serving.

St. John's Power®

St. John's Wort

 Nature's Herbs®

Each capsule contains: 250 mg certified potency St. John's wort extract concentrated and standardized for the preferred 0.14% hypericin, in a synergistic base of Wild countryside® St. John's wort powder.

As an occasional dietary supplement, take 1 capsule 3 times daily at mealtime.

Available in 60 capsules.

Internal use. Preservative-free.

Capsule.

Not recommended during pregnancy. People with fair skin should not overexpose themselves to strong sunlight while taking this product due to the photosensitizing nature of this plant.

St. John's Wort

Standardized

Albi Imports Ltd.

Each 460 mg capsule contains: St. John's wort standardized extract (0.3% Hypericin) 100 mg, St. John's wort powder 360 mg.

Take 1–3 capsules 1–2 hours before bed.

Available in 45, 90 and 180 capsules.

Internal use.

Capsule.

Do not use with alcohol. Consult with a health care professional if you are already taking antidepressants or Valium. May cause photosensitivity in some individuals when taken in large quantities.

St. John's Wort

A. Vogel

Bioforce AG

Contains: Alcohol, Fresh organically grown and wild St. John's wort herb.

Take 10-15 drops 3 times daily in small amount of water, 15 minutes before meals. Salivate before swallowing.

Available in 50 ml.

Internal use. Organic.

Tincture.

Exposure to sun while taking St. John's wort may cause skin irritations as the active ingredient, Hypericin, is a photosensitizing agent.

Not recommended during pregnancy.

St. John's Wort

0.3% Hypericin

naka Sales Ltd.

Each capsule contains: approx. 400 mg of: St. John's wort extract (Hypericum perforatum) 300 mg, St. John's wort herb 100 mg. Standardized to active substance 0.3% Hypericin in a shell containing gelatin and purified water.

Take 1 capsule 3 times daily with meal or as directed by a professional.

Available in 90 capsules.

Internal use.

Gelatin capsule.

Avoid excessive exposure to sunlight, tanning or UV sources.

St. John's Wort Extract

300 mg

Natural Factors® Nutritional Products Ltd.

Each capsule contains: St. John's wort extract (Hypericum perforatum) 300 mg, standardized to contain 0.3% Hypericin (900 mcg per capsule). Encapsulated in a gelatin capsule with vegetable grade Magnesium stearate (used as a lubricant).

Take 1 capsule in the evening.

Available in 90 capsules.

Internal use. Contains no artificial preservatives, color, dairy, sweeteners, starch, wheat or yeast.

Capsule.

Visual.

St. John's Wort Juice

W. Schoenenberger

Contains: Pure natural pressed herb and plant juice from

organically grown St. John's wort plants.

Shake bottle before use. Take 3 or 4 times daily before meals 1 tbsp. diluted in water, milk or tea, one part juice to six parts liquid. For children 1 tsp. full instead of tbsp. Unopened bottle will keep indefinitely: opened, for 6 days.

Amber bottle of 5.5 fl. oz.

Internal use. Organically grown in nearly ideal conditions in the Black Forest & Swabian uplands, where the air is pure. The plants are gathered at the moment when their production of valuable ingredients is at its peak. The juices are extracted by specially designed hydraulic presses that ensure maximum recovery of all essential elements, making certain that not more than 2-3 hours elapse between harvesting, pressing and bottling.

Cellular plant juice.

St. John's Wort Oil Extract

Flora Manufacturing & Distributing Ltd.

Each capsule contains: St. John's wort oil (Hypericum perforatum) extract 430 mg, derived from wild-crafted, organically grown St. John's wort blossoms (macerated in sunlight for 1000 hours) and Extra virgin olive oil.

Take 3-5 capsules daily with liquid for therapeutic and occasional use only.

Available in amber bottles of 90 and 180 capsules,

Internal use.

Capsule.

May cause drowsiness. Do not drive or engage in activities requiring alertness. Avoid alcoholic beverages. If taking this product, it is advisable to avoid long exposure to the sun and sun tanning beds.

Visual.

Star of Bethlehem
Bach Flower Remedy

Bach Flower Remedies® Ltd.

Contains: Ornithogalum umbellatum 5x in 27% grape alcohol solution.

Take 2 drops under the tongue 4 times daily or 2 drops in a small glass of spring water and sip at intervals.

10 ml with dropper.

Internal use.

Liquid.

Sting Gel
Homeopathic Cream

A. Nelson & Company Ltd.

Contains: Extracts of organically grown Pyrethrum pale 1x 3%, Ledum palustre 1x 1%, Arnica montana 1x 1%, Calendula officinalis 1x 1%, Rumex crispus 1x 1%, Echinacea purpurea 1x 1%, Hypericum perforatum 1x 1% in a water-soluble gel base.

Apply to bites and stings.

27 g tube.

External use. Organic. Not tested on animals.

Gel.

Avoid contact with eyes. If symptoms persist, consult a physician.

Stress B Formula
Plus 1000 mg C

Natural Factors® Nutritional Products Ltd.

Each tablet contains: Vitamin B-1 (Thiamine hydrochloride) 25 mg, Vitamin B-2 (Riboflavin) 25 mg, Niacinamide 25 mg, Vitamin B-6 (Pyridoxine hydrochloride) 25 mg, Vitamin B-12 (Cyanocobalamin) 25 mcg, Biotin 25 mcg, Folic acid 1 mg, d-Pantothenic acid 25 mg, Vitamin C 1000 mg. Lipotropic factors: Choline bitartrate 25 mg, Inositol 25 mg. Non-medicinal ingredients: Para Amino Benzoic acid 25 mg.

Take 1 tablet daily or as directed by a physician.

Available in 60 and 90 tablets.

Internal use. Contains no artificial preservatives, color, corn, dairy, gluten, soya, starch, sweeteners or yeast.

Tablet.

Visual.

Strix Bilberry Extract™

Scandinavian Natural Health & Beauty Products, Inc.

Each tablet contains: 80 mg of standardized Bilberry extract, (Vaccinium myrtillus) containing 25% anthocyanosides and 1 mg of Beta carotene in a base of Bilberry concentrate.

Take 2-6 tablets daily.

Available in blister packs of 30 and 60 tablets.

Internal use.

Tablet.

Sulphur
Homeopathic Remedy

A. Nelson & Company Ltd.

Each pillule contains: Sulphur 6c.

Take 2 pillules every 2 hours for the first 6 doses, then 4 times daily for up to 5 days. Pillules should be sucked or chewed and taken between meals.

84 pillules/globules per bottle.

Internal use.

Pillule/globule.

sunnie™

The Green Turtle Bay® Vitamin Co., Inc.

Each 4 caplets contains: Vitamins: C (as Niacorbate) 500 mg, B1 (as Thiamine) 10 mg, B2 (as Riboflavin) 10 mg, Niacin (as Niacinamide) 25 mg, B6 (as Pyridoxine) 10 mg, Folate (as Folic acid) 400 mcg, B12 (as Cyanocobalamin) 100 mcg, Biotin 50 mcg, d-Cal Pantothenate 50 mg, PABA 10 mg, Inositol 25 mg, Choline bitartrate 25 mg Minerals: Magnesium (as carbonate) 50 mg, Zinc (as monomethionate) 10 mg, Copper (glycinate) 0.5 mg, Manganese (as glycinate) 20 mg. Amino acids: L-glutamine 150 mg. Also contains: St. John's wort (0.3% hypericin), Hypericum perforatum L 900 mg, Betaine TMG 500 mg.

Take 2 tablets twice daily with food.

Available in bottles of 120 tablets.

Internal use.

Tablet.

May increase risk of sunburn.

Do not take with alcoholic beverages.

Super C 500 mg
Plus Rosehips & Bioflavonoids

Natural Factors® Nutritional Products Ltd.

Each tablet contains: Vitamin C 500 mg. Non-medicinal ingredients: Rosehips 500 mg, Lemon bioflavonoids 150 mg, Hesperidin 100 mg, Rutin 50 mg.

Take 1 tablet daily or as directed by a physician.

Available in 60, 90 and 180 tablets.

Internal use. Contains no artificial preservatives, color, dairy, sweeteners, starch, wheat or yeast.

Tablet.

Visual.

Super Glucosamine Sulfate

Albi Imports Ltd.

Each capsule contains: Glucosamine sulfate 500 mg or 1000 mg.

Take 1 capsule 3 times daily.

Available in 30, 60, 90 and 180 capsules.

Internal use.

Capsule.

Visual.

Super Multi
Iron Free

Natural Factors® Nutritional Products Ltd.

Each tablet contains: Beta carotene (Provitamin A) 10,000 IU, Vitamin D3 400 IU, Vitamin B-1 (Thiamine hydrochloride) 25 mg, Vitamin B-2 (Riboflavin) 25 mg, Niacinamide 50 mg, Vitamin B-6 (Pyridoxine hydrochloride) 25 mg, Vitamin B-12 (Cyanocobalamin) 50 mcg, Pantothenic acid (Calcium pantothenate) 25 mg, Folic acid 0.8 mg, Biotin 25 mcg,

Vitamin C (Ascorbic acid) 150 mg, Vitamin E (d-alpha Tocopheryl succinate) 50 IU. Lipotropic factors: Choline bitartrate 50 mg, Inositol 50 mg. Minerals: Calcium (citrate) 125 mg, Magnesium (citrate/oxide) 50 mg, Potassium (citrate) 10 mg, Zinc (citrate) 10 mg, Manganese (citrate) 5 mg, Iodine (kelp) 0.1 mg, Chromium (citrate) 100 mcg, Selenium (citrate) 20 mcg. Non-medicinal ingredients: Para Amino Benzoic acid 25 mg, Glutamic acid 25 mg.

Take 1 tablet daily or as directed by a physician.

Available in 60, 90 and 180 tablets.

Internal use. Contains no artificial preservatives, color, dairy, sweeteners, starch, wheat or yeast.

Tablet.

Visual.

Super Multi Plus

Natural Factors® Nutritional Products Ltd.

Each tablet contains: Beta carotene (Provitamin A) 10,000 IU, Vitamin A (Palmitate) 2500 IU, Vitamin D3 400 IU, Vitamin B-1 (Thiamine hydrochloride) 25 mg, Vitamin B-2 (Riboflavin) 25 mg, Niacinamide 50 mg, Vitamin B-6 (Pyridoxine hydrochloride) 25 mg, Vitamin B-12 (Cyanocobalamin) 50 mcg, Pantothenic acid (Calcium pantothenate) 25 mg, Folic acid 1 mg, Biotin 25 mcg, Vitamin C (Ascorbic acid)

150 mg, Vitamin E (d-alpha Tocopheryl succinate) 50 IU. Lipotropic factors: Choline bitartrate 50 mg, Inositol 50 mg. Minerals: Calcium (citrate/carbonate) 125 mg, Magnesium (citrate/oxide) 50 mg, Iron (citrate/fumerate) 10 mg, Potassium (citrate) 10 mg, Zinc (citrate) 10 mg, Manganese (citrate) 5 mg, Iodine (potassium/kelp) 0.1 mg, Chromium (HVP* chelate/citrate) 100 mcg, Selenium (HVP* chelate/citrate) 20 mcg. Non-medicinal ingredients: Para Amino Benzoic acid 25 mg, Citrus bioflavonoids 25 mg, Glutamic acid 25 mg, in a standard food extract base: Chlorella, organic Alfalfa, Barley grass, Carrot juice, Wheat grass juice, Broccoli extract. *Hydrolyzed vegetable protein (rice).

Take 1 tablet daily or as directed by a physician.

Available in 60, 90 and 180 tablets.

Internal use. Contains no artificial preservatives, color, dairy, sweeteners starch, gluten or yeast.

Tablet.

There is enough iron in this product to seriously harm a child.

Visual.

Super Once A Day

Quest Vitamins

Each tablet contains: Vitamin A (Palmitate) 10,000 IU, Vitamin D 400 IU, Vitamin E (d-alpha Tocopheryl acetate) 50 IU, Vitamin C (Ascorbic

acid) 150 mg, Vitamin B-1 (Thiamine hydrochloride) 50 mg, Vitamin B-2 (Riboflavin) 50 mg, Niacin 50 mg, Pantothenic acid (d-Calcium pantothenate) 50 mg, Vitamin B-6 (Pyridoxine hydrochloride) 50 mg, Folic acid 0.2 mg, Vitamin B-12 (Cobalamin conc.) 50 mcg, Biotin 50 mcg, Choline bitartrate 50 mg, Inositol 50 mg, Minerals: Calcium (HVP chelate, Calcium phosphate) 125 mg, Magnesium gluconate 100 mg, Phosphorus (HVP* chelate, Calcium phosphate) 50 mg, Potassium gluconate 50 mg, Iron (HVP* chelate) 15 mg, Zinc (HVP* chelate) 10 mg, Manganese (HVP* chelate) 1 mg, Copper (HVP* chelate) 1 mg, Iodine (Potassium iodide) 0.1 mg, Selenium (HVP* chelate) 25 mcg, Chromium (HVP* chelate) 25 mcg, Non-medicinal: PABA (Para amino benzoic acid) 50 mg, Citrus bioflavonoids 25 mg, Lecithin 15 mg, providing unsaturated fatty acids 6 mg, Betaine hydrochloride 12 mg, Hesperidin 10 mg, Papain 2 mg, Rutin 2 mg, L-cysteine 0.6 mg. *Hydrolyzed vegetable (rice) protein.

Take 1 tablet daily with morning or noon meal, or as directed by a health professional.

Available in 30, 60, 90 and 180 tablets per bottle.

Internal use. Each tablet is formulated to release gradually over a six hour period. CellCote coated tablet.

Tablet.

This product contains Niacin which may cause transient flushing and itching due to dilation of blood vessels and the release of Histamine.

Super Shape Citri-Plus

Maximum Strength

🏠 **Natural Factors® Nutritional Products Ltd.**

⚗️ Each capsule contains: (-)Hydroxycitric acid 50%, (-)HCA 500 mg (Garcinia cambogia), Bromelain 1000 GDU 100 mg, Grapefruit extract 50 mg, Pineapple extract 50 mg.

👐 Take 2-3 capsules daily or as directed by a physician.

📦 Available in 90 and 180 capsules.

Ⅱ Internal use. Contains no artificial preservatives, color, dairy, sweeteners, starch, wheat or yeast.

💊 Capsule.

📷 Visual.

Super Stress

Mega B Complex Plus C 1,000 mg

🏠 **Quest Vitamins**

⚗️ Each tablet contains: Vitamin C 1,000 mg, Vitamin B-1 (Thiamine hydrochloride) 50 mg, Vitamin B-2 (Riboflavin) 50 mg, Niacin 50 mg, Pantothenic acid (d-Calcium pantothenate) 50 mg, Vitamin B-6 (Pyridoxine hydrochloride) 50 mg, Folic acid 1 mg, Vitamin B-12 50 mcg, Biotin 50 mcg, Lipotropic factors: Choline bitartrate 50 mg, Inositol 50 mg. Non-medicinal Ingredients: PABA (Para amino Benzoic acid) 50 mg, Black cohosh root, Croscarmellose sodium, Hops, Ginger root, Magnesium stearate (vegetable source), Microcrystalline cellulose, Passion flower, Peppermint, Scullcap, Silicon dioxide, Valerian root, Vegetable stearin, Wood betony.

👐 Take 1 tablet daily or as directed by a physician.

📦 Available in 60 and 90 tablets.

Ⅱ Internal use. Easy-to-swallow CellCote coated tablet.

⊘ Tablet.

✋ This product contains Niacin which may cause transient flushing and itching due to dilation of blood vessels and the release of Histamine.

Swedish Bitters: Maria's Original Herbal Bitters

🏠 **Flora Manufacturing & Distributing Ltd.**

⚗️ Contains: Alcohol 39.4%, alcohol extracts of: Aloe (Aloe ferox) Angelica root (Angelica arch-angelica), Manna (Fraxinus ornus), Rhubarb root (Rheum palmatum) , Senna leaves (Cassia angustifolia), Zedvoary root (Curcuma zedoaria), Theriac venezian (Pimpinella saxifrago), Carline thistle root (Carlina acaulis), Myrrh (Commiphora molmol), Camphor (Cinnamomum camphora), Saffron (Crocus sativus).

👐 Shake the bottle well before using. Take 1 tsp. in water or herbal tea, 3-4 times daily.

📦 Available in amber bottles of 100 and 250 ml.

Ⅱ Internal and external use. Use within six weeks after opening.

💧 Liquid.

✋ Pregnant and lactating women should consult a qualified practioner before taking.

Swedish Bitters: Maria's Original Herbal Bitters

Alcohol Free

🏠 **Flora Manufacturing & Distributing Ltd.**

⚗️ Contains: Purified water, aqueous extracts of: Aloe (Aloe ferox) Angelica root (Angelica arch-angelica), Manna (Fraxinus ornus), Rhubarb root (Rheum palmatum) , Senna leaves (Cassia angustifolia), Zedvoary root (Curcuma zedoaria), Theriac venezian (Pimpinella saxifrago), Carline thistle root (Carlina acaulis), Myrrh (Commipbora molmol), Camphor (Cinnamomum campbora), Saffron (Crocus sativus).

👐 Shake the bottle well before using. Take 1 tbsp. in water or herbal tea, up to four times daily.

📦 Available in amber bottles of 100 and 250 ml.

Ⅱ Internal and external use. Use within six weeks after opening.

💧 Liquid.

✋ Pregnant and lactating women should consult a qualified practioner before taking.

Swedish Skin Gel

🏠 **Bio-Plex Products**

Contains: Pure apple cider vinegar, Vegetable glycerin, Extracts of Adonida, Aloe, Angelica root, Myrrh, Rhubarb, American saffron, Cherry bark, Speedwell and Zedoaira, Lubragel, Glydant.

Apply a small amount on affected area 2–3 times daily.

Available in 50 cc and 100 cc.

External use only. Not tested on animals.

Gel.

Sweet Chestnut

Bach Flower Remedy

Bach Flower Remedies® Ltd.

Contains: Castanea sativa 5x in 27% grape alcohol solution.

Take 2 drops under the tongue 4 times daily or 2 drops in a small glass of spring water and sip at intervals.

10 ml with dropper.

Internal use.

Liquid.

Tea Tree

Essential Oil

Bach-Karooch Ltd.

Contains: Melaleuca alternifolia 100%.

Two parts Essential oil must be diluted in 98 parts vegetable

oil before applying to the skin. Consult Aromatherapy literature for specific methods of use and directions for each oil.

10 ml in amber bottle with child-resistant cap and one-drop insert.

Oil.

Causes skin sensitivity in some individuals.

Caution: due to high concentration, all oils may be harmful if improperly used! External use only.

Tea Tree Oil Antiseptic Balm

Flora Herbal Cream

Flora Manufacturing & Distributing Ltd.

Contains: Distilled water, Tea tree oil, unrefined Flax oil (certified organic), Glyceryl stearate*, Glucose moisturizer, Glycerine, emulsifying wax, Phenonip (as cosmetic preservative), Lavender oil, Vitamin E. Tea tree oil content 3%. *Naturally derived from coconut.

Apply to affected area as needed. Wash hands after use.

60 ml in opaque jar.

External use. Use within 9 months of opening.

Balm.

Avoid contact with eyes.

TEETHA

Homeopathic Complex

A. Nelson & Company Ltd.

Each sachet contains: 6th homeopathic potency of Chamomilla.

Put the contents of 1 sachet into the child's mouth every 2 hours for up to 6 doses.

24 sachets.

Internal use.

Fine granules.

TEN-D-NIT POULTICE

Bio-Plex Products

Contains: Grey clay, Castor oil, Purified water, Lemon juice, Essential oils of Eucalyptus globulus and Lavender, Methylcellulose, Grapefruit seed extract, Germaben, Glydant.

Apply a thick coat on affected area. Cover with a sterilized cloth and leave on overnight. Repeat as needed.

Available in 250 cc and 1 litre.

External use only. Not tested on animals.

Paste.

The Ultimate Whey Designer Protein®

Next Nutrition

Contains: WPH (Vanilla praline flavor). Whey peptides [modified molecular weight and partially pre-digested (hydrolyzed) Whey protein concentrate], specially-filtered and new ion-exchanged Whey, Vanilla flavor, Lecithin, Praline extract, Vanilla extract, Cellulose gum, Xanthan gum, Malic acid, Annato (natural food coloring), Acesulfame-Potassium.

Mix 1-3 scoops in water or liquid and drink immediately. May be added to drinks, shakes, muffins, cereals, pancakes, waffles, sauces, yogurt.

Available in 22 g, 340 g and 907 g. Available in Vanilla-Praline, Chocolate and natural flavor.

Internal use. Mixes instantly.

Powder.

Visual.

Thistle Cleanse™

McZand® Herbal Inc.

Each capsule contains 100 mg of: Milk thistle extract (standardized to 80% silymarin) in a base of Milk thistle seed, Dandelion root, Yellow dock root, Dan shen root, Hyssop leaf, Red clover blossom, Burdock root, Barberry root, Bupleurum root, Sage leaf, Ginger root, Licorice root, Japanese honeysuckle flower and Chrysanthemum flower.

Take 1 or 2 capsules or 20–40 drops between meals 1 to 2 times daily.

Available in 59 ml liquid and 60 capsules.

Internal use.

Capsule.

Tincture.

Thuja
Homeopathic Remedy

A. Nelson & Company Ltd.

Each pillule contains: Thuja occidentalis 6c.

Take 2 pillules every 2 hours for the first 6 doses, then 4 times daily for up to 5 days. Pillules should be sucked or chewed and taken between meals.

84 pillules/globules per bottle.

Internal use.

Pillule/globule.

Thyme Red
Essential Oil

Bach-Karooch Ltd.

Contains: Thymus vulgaris 100%.

Two parts Essential oil must be diluted in 98 parts vegetable oil before applying to the skin. Consult Aromatherapy literature for specific methods of use and directions for each oil.

10 ml in amber bottle with child-resistant cap and one-drop insert.

Oil.

Can irritate mucous membranes and may cause skin irritation.

Caution: due to high concentration, all oils may be harmful if improperly used! External use only. Avoid during pregnancy.

Tomisal™

Biolinea GmbH

Contains: Pectin, Peppermint, Tannin, Calcium, Potassium chloride and Magnesium peroxide.

Apply once a day for 6 weeks.

Available in 250 ml.

External use only.

Cream.

Visual.

Traveler's Friend®

Nutribiotic

Contains: Grapefruit seed extract, Vegetable glycerin.

Available in 10 ml bottle.

Internal and external use.

Liquid.

Turmeric Power®

🏠 **Nature's Herbs®**

⚗️ Each capsule contains: 300 mg certified potency Turmeric extract concentrated and standardized for a minimum of preferred 95% curcumins, in a synergistic base of Turmeric powder.

✋ Take 1 capsule 2–3 times daily.

📦 Available in 60 capsules.

🔢 Internal use.

💊 Capsule.

Ubiquinone CoQ10 60 mg

🏠 **Flora Manufacturing & Distributing Ltd.**

⚗️ Each capsule contains: CoEnzyme Q10 (Ubiquinone) 60 mg in a base of powder of certified organically grown pre-cooked wild rice, in Vegicaps® (non-animal source, easily digested capsules).

✋ Take 1 or 2 capsules daily with meals.

📦 Available in 30 and 60 capsules.

🔢 Internal use only.

💊 Vegetarian capsule.

Udo's Choice Probiotics® Super Five

🏠 **Flora Manufacturing & Distributing Ltd.**

⚗️ Each tablet is guaranteed to contain: Not less than one billion total viable cells of: DDS-1™ Lactobacillus acidophilus 40%, NC-24 Bifidobacterium bifidum 15%, DDS-14 Lactobacillus bulgaricus 15%, NC-22 Streptococcus thermophilus 15%, NC-38 Lactobacillus salivarius 15%, in a base of Maltodextrin, Fructose and Ascorbic acid. With natural raspberry flavoring and natural coloring.

✋ Take 1-2 chewable tablets daily, one half hour before meals.

📦 Available in 60 tablets.

🔢 Internal use. Non-dairy. Ideal for traveling. For guaranteed potency, keep refrigerated.

🚫 Chewable tablet.

Udo's Choice® Ultimate Digestive Enzyme Blend

🏠 **Flora Manufacturing & Distributing Ltd.**

⚗️ Each 1000 mg capsule contains: 150 mg pure vegetable-source enzyme blend with guaranteed activity: Amylase 5000 DU, Protease 12500 HUT, Glucoamylase 4.5 AG, Malt diastase 270 DP, Pectinase (with Phytase)) 7.5 endo/PGU, Lipase 100 LU, Cellulase 400 CU, Invertase 0.2 IAU, Lactase 500 LacU, in a base of ground buckwheat powder; in Vegicaps® (vegetable fiber-source, high absorption capsules). All enzymes are expressed in accepted units of activity.

✋ Take 1 capsule at the beginning of a meal. For heavy meals: Take an additional capsule in the middle of the meal.

📦 Available in 90 capsules and travel packs of 21 capsules.

🔢 Internal use. A blend of nine vegetable-source enzymes. Compensates for the lack of enzymes in cooked or processed food. Contains 100% vegetable-source enzymes, in convenient Vegicaps®.

💊 Vegetarian capsule.

⚠️ Do not take on an empty stomach. May irritate existing ulcers. As enzymes are sensitive, it is advisable not to take them with high temperature foods such as soups, hot drinks or fried foods.

📷 Visual.

Udo's Choice® Ultimate Oil Blend®

🏠 **Flora Manufacturing & Distributing Ltd.**

⚗️ Each 250 ml contains: Flax oil, Sunflower oil, Sesame oil (from certified organically grown seeds), Medium chain triglycerides (MCT), Lecithin, Rice bran and Germ oils, oat bran and germ oils, d-alpha Tocopherol.

✋ Take 1 tbsp. 2 times daily with meals.

Available in 250 and 500 ml nitrogen-flushed amber bottles.

Cloudy layer is beneficial; shake gently before use. Keep refrigerated at all times, can be frozen to prolong freshness. Formulated by Udo Erasmus, author of Fats That Heal Fats That Kill. Mechanically pressed in a light and oxygen-free, low heat environment.

Oil.

Do not use for heating or frying foods.

Visual.

Udo's Choice® Ultimate Oil Blend®

Capsules

Flora Manufacturing & Distributing Ltd.

Each 1000 mg capsule contains: Flax oil, Sunflower oil, Sesame oil (made from certified organic flax, sesame and sunflower seeds), Medium chain triglycerides (MCT), Lecithin, Rice bran and Germ oils, Oat bran and Germ oils, d-alpha Tocopherol, in a gelatin capsule containing carob, from certified organically grown seeds. Added MCTs, Lecithin, Evening Primrose oil and Vitamin E. Contains unrefined oils from the germ of rice, oats and wheat.

Take 1-2 capsules 3 times daily with meals.

Available in 90 and 180 capsules of 1000 mg.

Internal use. In gelatin capsules containing carob to pro-

tect against light. Ideal for traveling. Mechanically pressed in a light and oxygen free, low heat environment. Formulated by Udo Erasmus, author of Fats that Heal Fats that Kill.

Capsule.

Visual.

Ultra Multi Plus

with Mineral Citrate Complex

 Natural Factors® Nutritional Products Ltd.

Each tablet contains: Beta carotene (Provitamin A) 10,000 IU, Vitamin A (palmitate) 2500 IU, Vitamin D3 (Lanolin) 400 IU, Lanolin, Vitamin B-1 (Thiamine hydrochloride) 50 mg, Vitamin B-2 (Riboflavin/riboflavin '5' phosphate) 50 mg, Vitamin B-3 (Niacin) 10 mg, Niacinamide 50 mg, Vitamin B-6 (Pyridoxine pyridoxal '5' phosphate) 50 mg, Vitamin B-12 (Cobalamin) 100 mcg, Pantothenic acid (Calcium pantothenate) 50 mg, Folic acid 0.8 mg, Biotin 50 mcg, Vitamin C (Calcium ascorbate) 150 mg, Vitamin E (d-alpha Tocopheryl succinate) 100 IU. Lipotropic factors: Choline bitartrate 50 mg, Inositol 50 mg, Methionine 50 mg. Minerals: Calcium (citrate/carbonate) 125 mg, Magnesium (citrate/oxide) 75 mg, Iron (citrate/fumerate) 10 mg, Manganese (citrate) 5 mg, Potassium (citrate) 50 mg, Zinc (citrate) 12 mg, Iodine (Potassium/kelp) 0.1 mg, Chromium (HVP* chelate) 50 mcg, Molybdenum (citrate) 50 mcg, Selenium (HVP* chelate) 50 mcg. Non-medicinal: Para Amino Benzoic acid 50 mg, Citrus bioflavonoids 25

mg, Betaine hydrochloride 30 mg, Bromelain 25 mg, Kelp 10 mg, Vanadium (citrate) 100 mcg in a standard food extract base: Chlorella, organic Alfalfa, Barley grass juice, Carrot juice, Wheat grass juice, Broccoli extract. *Hydrolyzed vegetable protein (rice).

Take 1 tablet daily or as directed by a physicians.

Available in 60, 90 and 180 tablets.

Internal use. Contains no artificial preservatives, color, dairy, sweeteners starch, gluten or yeast.

Tablet.

There is enough iron in this product to seriously harm a child.

Visual.

Ultra Prim Primrose Oil

1000 mg

Natural Factors® Nutritional Products Ltd.

Each capsule contains: Gamma-linolenic acid 100 mg, Cis-linoleic acid 720 mg (from 1000 mg of evening primrose oil), Vitamin E (d-alpha Tocopherol) 30 IU.

Take 2-3 capsules daily or as directed by a physician.

Available in 60, 90, 180 and 360 softgel capsules.

Internal use. Contains no artificial preservatives, color, dairy, sweeteners, starch, wheat or yeast.

Softgel capsule.

Visual.

Ultra Prim Primrose Oil 500 mg

Natural Factors® Nutritional Products Ltd.

Each capsule contains: Gamma-linolenic acid 50 mg, Cis-linoleic acid 360 mg (from 500 mg of Evening Primrose oil) Vitamin E (d-alpha tocopherol) 14.9 IU.

Take 3-6 capsules daily or as directed by a physician.

Available in 60, 90, 180 and 360 softgel capsules.

Internal use. Naturally press-extracted at low temperature without solvents.

Softgel capsule.

Visual.

Ultra-Gar™
Organic Garlic

Prairie Naturals®

Each 500 mg capsule contains: Alliin rich garlic powder, organic Chinese garlic (contains not less than) alliin 50 mg. Total sulphur compounds 50 mg (s-allyl mercaptocysteine, di-allyl sulphide, methyl-allyl-sulphide).

Take 1-3 capsules daily with meals.

Available 180 capsules.

Internal use. Contains no artificial preservatives, color, flavors, starch, dairy, yeast or gluten.

Capsule.

Visual.

Ultra-Sil
Spring Horsetail Extract

Prairie Naturals®

Each 500 mg capsule contains: Aqueous extract of Spring horsetail (Equisetum arvense) equivalent to 15 mg of the most concentrated and bioavailable (organic) vegetal Silica. Synergistically formulated with Norwegian kelp powder, a natural source of important trace minerals.

Take 1-4 capsules daily with meals or as directed by a physician.

Available in 30, 90 and 180 capsules.

Internal use. Prairie Naturals® Spring Horsetail™ (Equesetum arvense) is known to contain: Silica, Flavonoids, Manganese, Potassium, Sulphur, Magnesium, Calcium, Iron and Phosphorous. Free of yeast, gluten, starch, soya, egg, dairy, artificial color, preservatives, solvents or alcohol.

Capsule.

Visual.

Uncle Lee's Green Teas®

Uncle Lee's Teas® Inc.

Contains: Green tea leaves. May also contain natural flavors.

Available in 20 tea bag box size. Herbal Tea. Also available in regular, tropical fruit, cinnamon apple.

Internal use. Green tea does contain some caffeine, about 1/3 the amount of a cup of coffee.

Herbal Tea.

Those people extremely sensitive to caffeine should consider avoiding this product.

Visual.

Urticalcin®
A. Vogel
Homeopathic Remedy

Bioforce AG

Contains: Calcarea carbonica 4x, Calcarea phosphorica 6x, Natrum phosphoricum 6x, Silicea 6x, Urtica dioica 1x.

Take 2 tablets under the tongue, 3 times daily 15 minutes before meals.

Available in 400 tablets.

Internal use.

Tablet.

Uva Ursi Leaf

Nature's Herbs®

Each 505 mg capsule contains: Wild countryside® Uva ursi (Bearberry) leaf.

Take 1-3 capsules 3 times daily with a full glass of water preferably at mealtimes.

Available in 100 capsules.

Internal use. Preservative-free.

Capsule.

Valerian Tincture

Salus-Haus

Each 10 g tincture contains: 10 g extract derived from 2.0 g Valerian roots.

Unless otherwise directed, take 15-20 drops diluted in a small amount of liquid 3 to 4 times daily.

Available in 50 ml, includes a dropper.

Internal use. Salus herbal tinctures are made in accordance with strictest health food principles, using natural ingredients only.

Tincture.

Valerian-Power®

Nature's Herbs®

Each 455 mg capsule contains: 250 mg Certified potency Valerian root extract, concentrated and standardized for a minimum of preferred 0.8% valerenic acids, in a synergistic base of Wild countryside® Valerian root.

Take1-2 capsules twice daily with a full glass of water or 3-4 capsules 30 minutes before bedtime.

Available in 60 capsules.

Internal use. Preservative-free.

Capsule.

Do not use when driving a motor vehicle or operating machinery. Do not use if you are taking sedatives or tranquilizers without first consulting a health care professional.

Verbena (lemon)
Essential Oil

Bach-Karooch Ltd.

Contains: Lippia citriodora 100%.

Two parts Essential oil must be diluted in 98 parts vegetable oil before applying to the skin. Consult Aromatherapy literature for specific methods of use and directions for each oil.

10 ml in amber bottle with child-resistant cap and one-drop insert.

Oil.

Possible sensitization; possible phototoxicity.

Caution: due to high concentration, all oils may be harmful if improperly used! External use only.

Vervain
Bach Flower Remedy

Bach Flower Remedies® Ltd.

Contains: Verbena officinalis 5x in 27% grape alcohol solution.

Take 2 drops under the tongue 4 times daily or 2 drops in a small glass of spring water and sip at intervals.

10 ml with dropper.

Internal use.

Liquid.

Vetivert
Essential Oil

Bach-Karooch Ltd.

Contains: Vetiveria zizanoides 100%.

Two parts Essential oil must be diluted in 98 parts vegetable oil before applying to the skin. Consult Aromatherapy literature for specific methods of use and directions for each oil.

10 ml in amber bottle with child-resistant cap and one-drop insert.

Oil.

Caution: due to high concentration, all oils may be harmful if improperly used! External use only.

Vine

Bach Flower Remedy

🏠 **Bach Flower Remedies® Ltd.**

⚗️ Contains: Vitis vinifera 5x in 27% grape alcohol solution.

✋ Take 2 drops under the tongue 4 times daily or 2 drops in a small glass of spring water and sip at intervals.

📦 10 ml with dropper.

🔲 Internal use.

💧 Liquid.

Vital-Hair Multi Vitamin Supplement

🏠 **Life-Time Nutrition Inc.**

⚗️ Each tablet contains: Vitamin A 5,000 IU, Vitamin C 300 mg, Thiamine 15 mg, Riboflavin 15 mg, Niacinamide 15 mg, Pyridoxine hydrochloride 15 mg, Pantothenic acid 250 mg, Folic acid 0.4 mg, Biotin 1,000 mcg, Zinc 2.5 mg. Lipotropic factors: Choline 15 mg, Inositol 300 mg. Non-medicinal ingredients: L-Cysteine 100 mg, Para-amino Benzoic acid 100 mg.

✋ Take 1 tablet daily or as directed by a physician.

📦 Available in 60 capsules.

🔲 Internal use.

💊 Capsule.

📷 Visual.

Vital-Plex

🏠 **Klaire Laboratories, Inc., USA & Europe**

⚗️ Each capsule contains: Lactobacillus acidophilus DDS-1™ 1 billion PLUS, Bifidobacterium bifidum 1 Billion PLUS, Streptococcus faecium 1 Billion PLUS. Additional ingredients are proprietary as per Nebraska Cultures. The dark specks in this formulation are natural stabilizers and enhance this product.

✋ Take 1 or 2 capsules with food daily or as directed by a physician.

📦 Available in 100 capsules.

🔲 Internal use. A Non-dairy combination of microorganisms. Because Vital-Plex is free of milk, soy, MSG, yeast and other common allergens, it is well tolerated by even the most allergic individual.

💊 Capsule.

Vitamin C 1000 mg

Plus Bioflavonoids and Rosehips

🏠 **Natural Factors® Nutritional Products Ltd.**

⚗️ Each tablet contains: Vitamin C 1000 mg. Non-medicinal ingredients: Citrus bioflavonoids 100 mg, Rosehips 100 mg.

✋ Take 1 tablet daily or as directed by a physician.

📦 Available in 60, 90, 180 and 360 tablets.

🔲 Internal use. Contains no artificial preservatives, color, dairy, sweeteners, starch, wheat or yeast.

⊘ Tablet.

📷 Visual.

Vitamin C 1000 mg

Time Release

🏠 **Natural Factors® Nutritional Products Ltd.**

⚗️ Each tablet contains: Vitamin C 1000 mg. Non-medicinal ingredients: Citrus bioflavonoids 200 mg.

✋ Take 1 tablet daily or as directed by a physicians.

📦 Available in 60, 90, 180 and 360 tablets.

🔲 Internal use. Time released tablets are designed to gradually release their contents over an eight hour period. Contains no artificial preservatives, color, dairy, sweeteners, starch, wheat or yeast.

⊘ Tablet.

📷 Visual.

Vitamin C 1500 mg

Time Release

🏠 **Natural Factors® Nutritional Products Ltd.**

⚗️ Each tablet contains: Vitamin C 1500 mg. Non-medicinal ingredients: Citrus bioflavonoids 200 mg.

✋ Take 1 tablet daily or as directed by a physician.

Available in 60 and 90 tablets.

Internal use. Time released tablets are designed to gradually release their contents over an eight hour period. Contains no artificial preservatives, color, dairy, sweeteners, starch, wheat or yeast.

Tablet.

Visual.

Vitamin E
Natural Ratio

Quest Vitamins

Each capsule contains: Vitamin E (d-alpha Tocopherol) 400 IU. Non-medicinal ingredients: 67 mg each of d-beta Tocopherol, d-delta Tocopherol, d-gamma Tocopherol. Derived from natural vegetable oils with wheat germ oil.

Take 1 capsule daily, or as directed by a health professional.

Available in 90 and 180 capsules.

Internal use. Contains no artificial preservatives, color, flavors or added sugar, starch, milk products or yeast.

Capsule.

Walnut
Bach Flower Remedy

Bach Flower Remedies® Ltd.

Contains: Juglans regia 5x in 27% grape alcohol solution.

Take 2 drops under the tongue 4 times daily or 2 drops in a small glass of spring water and sip at intervals.

10 ml with dropper.

Internal use.

Liquid.

Water Violet
Bach Flower Remedy

Bach Flower Remedies® Ltd.

Contains: Hottonia palustris 5x in 27% grape alcohol solution.

Take 2 drops under the tongue 4 times daily or 2 drops in a small glass of spring water and sip at intervals.

10 ml with dropper.

Internal use.

Liquid.

White Chestnut
Bach Flower Remedy

Bach Flower Remedies® Ltd.

Contains: Aesculus hippocastanum 5x in 27% grape alcohol solution.

Take 2 drops under the tongue 4 times daily or 2 drops in a small glass of spring water and sip at intervals.

10 ml with dropper.

Internal use.

Liquid.

White Lightning™ Hair and Scalp Revitalizing Formula

Prairie Naturals®

Contains: Cold Pressed Virgin Olive Oil, Herbal Extracts of Rosemary, Mullein, Cherry Bark, Nettle, Yarrow, Marshmallow Root, Comfrey, Oak Bark, Black Walnut, Chickweed and Spring Horsetail, Essential Oil of Eucalyptus, Rosemary, Clary Sage and Basil, Polysorbate 80, Jojoba Oil, Biotin, Niacin, Folic Acid, Vitamin E Oil, Cystine/Cysteine, Grapefruit Seed Extract.

Massage 20 drops into the scalp. Leave on overnight as a treatment to promote the proper functioning of hair follicles.

Available in 125 ml dropper bottles.

External use only. Enviro-wise and biodegradable. Not tested on animals.

Liquid.

White Oak

Nature's Herbs®

Each 430 mg capsule contains: White oak bark, gelatin.

 Take 3 capsules 3 times daily with a large glass of water.

Available in 100 capsules.

Internal use.

Capsule.

White Willow

Nature's Herbs®

Each 379 mg capsule contains Wild Countryside® White willow bark.

Take 2-3 capsules every three hours as needed up to 18 capsules per day.

100 capsules.

Internal use. Preservative-free.

Capsule.

Wild Alaskan Salmon Oil
1000 mg

Natural Factors® Nutritional Products Ltd.

Each capsule contains: Wild Alaskan salmon oil 1000 mg.

Take 1 to 2 capsules daily or as directed by a physicians.

Available in 90 and 180 softgel capsules.

Internal use. Contains no artificial preservatives, color, dairy, starch, wheat or yeast. Natural factors supports the sustainable use of wild salmon through contributions to the Pacific salmon foundation. This product is a value added by-product from the wild salmon fishery. The oil is extracted from already harvested wild salmon using fish parts that would otherwise be wasted.

Softgel capsule.

Visual.

Wild Oat
Bach Flower Remedy

Bach Flower Remedies® Ltd.

Contains: Bromus ramosus 5x in 27% grape alcohol solution.

Take 2 drops under the tongue 4 times daily or 2 drops in a small glass of spring water and sip at intervals.

10 ml with dropper.

Internal use.

Liquid.

Wild Rose
Bach Flower Remedy

Bach Flower Remedies® Ltd.

Contains: Rosa canina 5x in 27% grape alcohol solution.

Take 2 drops under the tongue 4 times daily or 2 drops in a small glass of spring water and sip at intervals.

10 ml with dropper.

Internal use.

Liquid.

Wild Rose Di-gest™

Wild Rose Laboratories

Each capsule contains: Glutamic acid HCI 100 mg, Betaine HCI 100 mg, Calcium ascorbate 50 mg, Pancreatin N.F. 360 mg, Bromelain 1:10 80 mg, Papain 75 mg.

Take 3 to 4 capsules during meals, or as recommended by your physician or qualified health practitioner.

Available in 60 and 150 capsules.

Internal use. Formulated by Dr. Terry Willard, PhD, Master Herbalist.

Capsule.

Contraindicated for stomach ulcers.

Wild Rose Femaherb™

Wild Rose Laboratories

Each tablet contains: Dong quai 172 mg in a base of Black cohosh, Blue cohosh, Blessed thistle, Cramp bark.

Take 1 or more tablets as desired, at mealtime with water or prepared as a tea.

Available in 100 and 250 tablets.

Internal use. Formulated by Dr. Terry Willard, PhD., Master Herbalist.

Tablet.

Do not consume Dong quai or Black cohosh during pregnancy.

Wild Rose Herbal D-Tox 12 Day Kit™

Wild Rose Laboratories

Contains: Four Wild Rose formulations: Biliherb, Laxaherb, Cleansaherb, CL herbal extract.

Take 2 tablets from each bottle of Biliherb, Laxaherb, and Cleansaherb with both breakfast and supper for 12 days. Take 2 full droppers (20 drops) of CL herbal extract during breakfast and supper for 12 days.

12 day program, boxed kit.

Internal use. Formulated by Dr. Terry Willard, PhD., Master Herbalist.

Tablet.

Tincture.

Wild Rose LBT 3™

Lower Bowel Tonic

Wild Rose Laboratories

Contains: Cascara Sagrada, Buckthorn, Ground raspberry, Ginger root, Red raspberry leaf, Fennel seed, Turkey rhubarb, Cayenne pepper.

Take 1 or more tablets as desired, at mealtime with water or prepared as tea.

Available in 100 and 250 tablets.

Internal use. Formulated by Dr. Terry Willard, Ph. D., Master Herbalist.

Tablet.

Wild Rose Respaherb™

Wild Rose Laboratories

Each tablet contains: Mao 180 mg, Reishi 60 mg, Elecampane root 60 mg, Ginger root, Mullein leaf.

Take 1 or more tablets as desired, at mealtime (3 times daily) with water or prepared as a tea.

Available in 100 and 250 tablets.

Internal use. Formulated by Dr. Terry Willard, Ph. D., Master Herbalist.

Tablet.

In cases of high blood pressure or heart disease, this formula should only be used under supervision of a qualified health practitioner.

Willow

Bach Flower Remedy

Bach Flower Remedies® Ltd.

Contains: Salix vitallina 5x in 27% grape alcohol solution.

Take 2 drops under the tongue 4 times daily or 2 drops in a small glass of spring water and sip at intervals.

10 ml with dropper.

Internal use.

Liquid.

Willowprin®

Nature's Herbs®

Two capsules contain: Certified potency White willow bark extract 200 mg, concentrated and standardized at 15% salicin (a natural constituent), equivalent to about 4000 mg of dry White willow bark, White willow bark 5:1 500 mg, equivalent to 2500 mg of White willow. White willow bark 200 mg.

Take 2-3 capsules every 4 hours as desired up to 18 capsules per day.

Available in 30 capsules.

Internal use. Preservative-free.

Capsule.

XtraPure™ Cynarol™ Artichoke

Complete Plant Concentrate 1:11

Dr. Dunner AG

Each capsule contains: Artichoke (Cynara scolymus)

plant concentrate (flower buds) 500 mg guaranteed equivalent to 5500 mg of pure artichoke in a base of Soybean oil, Beta-carotene (for color); in a softgel capsule (gelatin, glycerol, water).

Take 4 capsules throughout the day with liquid, unless otherwise indicated. A course of capsules should be taken for at least 12 weeks.

Available in 40 capsules blisterpacked.

Internal use. Guaranteed no additives or processing residues.

Softgel capsule.

Yarrow Flowers

Nature's Herbs®

Each 340 mg capsule contains: Yarrow flowers.

Take 2 capsules 2-3 times daily, preferably with meals.

Available in 100 capsules.

Internal use.

Capsule.

Yarrow Tincture

Salus-Haus

Each 10 g tincture contains: 10 g extract derived from 2 g of Yarrow blossoms.

Unless otherwise directed, take 10-20 drops before meals diluted in a small amount of liquid.

Available in 50 ml, includes a dropper.

Internal use.

Tincture.

Yeast Busters Program

Inno-Vite Inc.

The Yeast buster kit contains: Caproil (Caprylic acid and olive oil) 500 ml, 100% Psyllium husks and seed powder 280 g, DDS acidophilus 2.5 oz, Bentonite (Purified water, Bentonite).

Mix all ingredients together with water. Take once or twice daily on an empty stomach.

Products sold separately or together in kit.

Internal use.

Liquid.

Powder.

Some women may experience a change in menstrual cycle.

Do not use in the presence of nausea, vomiting or abdominal pain. Do not take within 2 hours of other medicines. Do not take if you have a Psyllium allergy. Avoid inhalation of Psyllium.

Visual.

Yellow Dock Root

Nature's Herbs®

Each 505 mg capsule contains: Wild countryside® Yellow dock root.

Take 2-3 capsules 3 times daily with a full glass of water.

Available in 100 capsules.

Internal use. Preservative-free.

Capsule.

Ylang-Ylang
Essential Oil

Bach-Karooch Ltd.

Contains: Cananga odorata 100%.

Two parts Essential oil must be diluted in 98 parts vegetable oil before applying to the skin. Consult Aromatherapy literature for specific methods of use and directions for each oil.

10 ml in amber bottle with child-resistant cap and one-drop insert.

Oil.

Can cause headaches or nausea; use in moderation.

Caution: due to high concentration, all oils may be harmful if improperly used! External use only.

Yucca

Nature's Herbs®

Each capsule contains: Wild countryside® Yucca stalk 490 mg.

Take 3 capsules 3 times daily with a large glass of water.

Available in 100 capsules.

Internal use. Preservative-free.

Capsule.

Zinc Citrate

50 mg

Natural Factors® Nutritional Products Ltd.

Each tablet contains: elemental Zinc (citrate) 50 mg. Non-medicinal ingredient: Sodium alginate 15 mg.

Take 1 tablet daily, preferably with meals or as directed by a physician.

Available in 90 and 180 tablets.

Internal use. Contains no artificial preservatives, color, dairy, sweeteners, starch, wheat or yeast.

Tablet.

Visual.

Zinc Plus

Klaire Laboratories, Inc., USA & Europe

Each capsule contains: Vitamin C (Ascorbic acid) 60 mg, Zinc (Zinc citrate) 15 mg, Vitamin B6 (Pyridoxine HCl) 4 mg. Added ingredients: Cellulose and L-leucine.

Take 1 capsule daily or as directed by a physician.

Available in 60 capsules.

Internal use. Highly soluble.

Capsule.

Zinc & Vitamin C Lozenges

Quest Vitamins

Each lozenge contains: Zinc (gluconate) 10 mg, Vitamin C (Ester C® brand Calcium ascorbate) 100 mg. Non-medicinal Ingredients: Echinacea angustifolia 55 mg (provided by 8 mg PE 1:7). Natural honey lemon flavor, Astragalus root, Chamomile flower, Red raspberry leaf, Peppermint leaf, Ginger root, Citric acid, Magnesium stearate, Silicon dioxide, Sorbitol, Sucralose.

Dissolve in mouth or chew 1 lozenge every 2 hours, to a maximum of 5 lozenges daily, or as directed by a health professional.

Available in 30 lozenges blister packed.

Lozenges. Contains no artificial preservatives, colors, flavoring or added sugar, starch, milk products, wheat, yeast, or animal substances.

Manufacturer and Distributor Listings

Section II

Manufacturers are listed alphabetically and identified by the color blue.
Immediately following each manufacturer are their worldwide distributors.

A. Nelson & Company Ltd.
Broadheath House
83 Parkside, London,
United Kingdom
SW19 5LP
Tel: 0181 780-4200
Fax: 0181 789-0275

Bach-Karooch Ltd.
P.O. Box 2465
Peterborough, ON
Canada
K9J 7Y8
Tel: (705) 749-1894
Fax: (705) 749-0275
e-mail:
wildboy@peterboro.net

Nelson Bach USA, Ltd.
Wilmington Technology Park
100 Research Drive
Wilmington, MA
USA
01887-4406
Tel: (508) 988-3833
Fax: (508) 988-0233

Albi Imports Ltd.
15-8980 Fraserwood Court
Burnaby, BC
Canada
V5J 5H7
Tel: (604) 438-1054
Fax: (604) 438-2029

Albi Imports
1122 Fir Avenue
Blaine, WA
USA
98230
Tel: (206) 575-8010
Fax: (206) 575-3141
Toll-free: 1-800-316-7517

Alvin Last, Inc.
19 Babcock Place
Yonkers, NY
USA
10701
Tel: (914) 376-1000
Fax: (914) 376-1001

Purity Life Health
Products Ltd.
6 Commerce Crescent
Acton, ON
Canada
L7J 2X3
Tel: (519) 853-3511
Fax: (519) 853-4660
Toll-free: 1-800-265-2615

Cornucopia Natural Foods
260 Lake Road
Dayville, CT
USA
06241
Tel: (860) 779-2807
Fax: (860) 779-2811

Tree of Life SE
4055 Deerpark Blvd.
Elkton, FL
USA
32033
Fax: (904) 825-2012
Toll-free: 1-800-874-0851

Food For Health
3655 W. Washington Street
Phoenix, AZ
USA
85009
Tel: (602) 269-2371
Fax: (602) 352-7553

Nature's Best
105 S. Puente Street
Brea, CA
USA
92262
Tel: (714) 441-2378
Fax: (714) 441-2330

Radiant Technologies
12 Atholl Road
Elton Hill, Johannesburg
South Africa
2196
Tel: 2711 440-4477
Fax: 2711 440-4477

Victoria Health
23 Broadwalk Shopping Centre
Edgware, Middlesex
England
HA8 7PD
Tel: 0181 905-6931
Fax: 0181 905-6931

Anton Huebner GmbH
& CO KG
Schloss Str. 11-17
Ehrenkirchen
Germany
D-79238
Tel:++49 7633 9090
Fax: ++49 7633 909240

naka Sales Ltd.
53 Queen's Plate Drive
Etobicoke, ON
Canada
M9W 6P1
Tel: (416) 748-3073
Fax: (416) 748-1555

Abkit Inc.
207 E. 94th
New York, NY
USA
10128
Tel: (212) 860 8358
Fax: (212) 860 8323

Medical Supplies
International
Excor Office Park
Bosbok Road
Randpark Ridge
South Africa
2156
Tel: ++27 11 791 0927
Fax: ++27 11 791 0935

Silicea Australia
9 Humphries Road
Frankston
Australia
3199
Tel: ++61 3 9787 0091
Fax: ++61 3 9787 0091

Red Seal Natural Health Ltd.
46 Honan Place
P.O. Box 19-046
Avondale, Aukland 7
New Zealand
Tel: ++64 9 828 0036
Fax: ++64 9 828 2499

Nature Works Co.
Room 603, David House
8-20 Nanking Street
Kowloon
Hong Kong
Tel: ++852 2782 1978
Fax: ++852 2782 1722

Artesian Acres Inc.
RR #3
Lacombe, AB
Canada
T0C 1S0
Tel: (403) 782-5075
Fax: (403) 782-5334

Aubrey Organics®
4416 N. Manhattan Avenue
Tampa, FL
USA
33614
Tel: (813) 877-4186
Fax: (813) 876-8166

New Age Marketing
14757 Upper Roper Road
White Rock, BC
Canada
V4B 2E1
Fax: (813) 876-8166
Toll-free: 1-888-868-0128

Bach Flower Remedies® Ltd.
Unit 6, Suffolk Way
Abingdon, Oxon
United Kingdom
0X14 SJX
Tel: 01235 550086
Fax: 01235 523973

Bach-Karooch Ltd.
P.O. Box 2465
Peterborough, ON
Canada
K9J 7Y8
Tel: (705) 749-1894
Fax: (705) 749-0275
e-mail:
wildboy@peterboro.net

Nelson Bach USA, Ltd.
Wilmington Technology Park
100 Research Drive
Wilmington, MA
USA
01887-4406
Tel: (508) 988-3833
Fax: (508) 988-0233

Bach-Karooch Ltd.
572 Neal Drive
Peterborough, ON
Canada
K9J 6X7
Tel: (705) 749-1894
Fax: (705) 749-0275

Bee Health Propolis
Racecourse Road, E. Ayton
Scarborough, N. Yorkshire
England
Y013 9HT
Tel:44 1723 864 001
Fax: 44 1723 862455

Inno-Vite Inc.
196 Wildcat Road
Downsview, ON
Canada
M3J 2N5
Tel: (416) 661-8272
Fax: (416) 661-5992

Bio-K+™ International Inc.
1155 Rue Metcalfe
Montreal, QC
Canada
H3B 2V6
Tel: (514) 954-1724
Fax: (514) 395-8780

Greens+ Canada
689 Queen Street W.
Toronto, ON
Canada
M6J 1E6
Tel: (416) 977-3505
Fax: (416) 977-4184
Toll-free: 1-800-258-0444

Bio-Plex Products
266 RR #1
Nedelec, QC
Canada
J0Z 2Z0
Tel: (819) 784-5411
Fax: (819) 784-2120

Bio-Strath AG®
Postfach 76
Roggwil TG
Switzerland
Tel:++41 71 454-6161
Fax: ++41 71 454-6162

Bioforce Canada Inc.
4001 Cote Vertu
St. Laurent, QC
Canada
H4R 1R5
Tel: (514) 335-9393
Fax: (514) 335-9639

Bioforce of America
122 Smith Road Extension
P.O. Box 507
Kinderhook, NY
USA
12106
Tel: (518) 758-6060
Fax: (518) 758-9500

Bioforce AG
Mühlebachstrasse 25
Zurich
Switzerland
CH-8032
Tel:++41 1 251-81-51
Fax: ++41 1 262-43-26

Bioforce Canada Inc.
4001 Cote Vertu
St. Laurent, QC
Canada
H4R 1R5
Tel: (514) 335-9393
Fax: (514) 335-9639

Bioforce of America
122 Smith Road Extension
P.O. Box 507
Kinderhook, NY
USA
12106
Tel: (518) 758-6060
Fax: (518) 758-9500

Biolina GmbH
Erdinger 14
Aschheim
Germany
D-85609
Tel:++49 89 945 524 40
Fax: ++49 89 945 524 21

Teldon of Canada Ltd.
7432 Fraser Park Drive
Burnaby, BC
Canada
V5J 5B9
Tel: (604) 436-0545
Fax: (604) 435-4862
Toll-free: 1-800-663-2212

Bodywise (UK) Ltd.
14 Lower Court Road
Lower Almondsbury, Bristol
England
BS12 4DX
Tel: 44 1454 615500
Fax: 44 1454 613805

Inno-Vite Inc.
196 Wildcat Road
Downsview, ON
Canada
M3J 2N5
Tel: (416) 661-8272
Fax: (416) 661-5992

Börner GmbH
Moosrosen Str. 7-13
Berlin
Germany
12347
Tel:++30 600-0010
Fax: ++30 606-1085

Life-Time Nutrition Inc.
Unit #107
12414-82nd Avenue
Surrey, BC
Canada
V3W 3E9
Tel: (604) 597-8050
Fax: (604) 597-6968

Dr. Dunner AG
Switzerland

Flora Manufacturing and
Distributing Ltd.
7400 Fraser Park Drive
Burnaby, BC
Canada
V5J 5B9
Tel: (604) 436-6000
Fax: (604) 436-6060

EAS
555 Corporate Circle
Golden, CO
USA
80401
Tel: (303) 384-0080
Fax: (303) 279-6465

Upper 49th Imports
1463 Dugald Road
Winnipeg, MB
Canada
R2J 0H3
Tel: (204) 233-3132
Fax: (204) 237-7019
Toll-free: 1-800-563-0965

**Efamol Research
Institute**
15 Chipman Drive
Kentville, NS
Canada
B4N 4H8
Tel: (902) 678-5534
Fax: (902) 678-9440

Flora Manufacturing and
Distributing Ltd.
7400 Fraser Park Drive
Burnaby, BC
Canada
V5J 5B9
Tel: (604) 436-6000
Fax: (604) 436-6060

Essiac International
164 Richmond Road
Ottawa, ON
Canada
K1Z 6W2
Call for a distributor near you:
(613) 729-9111

**Evergreen Wheatgrass
Juices Inc.**
P.O. Box #1
Don Mills, ON
Canada
M3C 2R6
Call for a distributor near you:
(905) 709-2770

Horizon Distributors
8335 Winston Street
Burnaby, BC
Canada
V5A 2H3
Tel: (604) 420-6751
Fax: (604) 420-0178

Timbuktu Natural Foods
2-752 Cochrane Drive
Markham, ON
Canada
L3R 8E1
Tel: (905) 477-7755
Fax: (905) 477-7761
Toll-free: 1-800-668-6518

Jelian Distributors Inc.
15 Connie Crescent, Unit 23
Concord, ON
Canada
L4K 1L3
Tel: (905) 660-0093
Fax: (905) 660-0390

F. Trenka
Austria

Flora Manufacturing and
Distributing Ltd.
7400 Fraser Park Drive
Burnaby, BC
Canada
V5J 5B9
Tel: (604) 436-6000
Fax: (604) 436-6060

Flora Manufacturing and Distributing Ltd.
7400 Fraser Park Drive
Burnaby, BC
Canada
V5J 5B9
Tel: (604) 436-6000
Fax: (604) 436-6060

Flora Inc.
Box 73, East Badger Road
Lynden, WA
USA
98264
Tel: (360) 354-2110
Fax: (360) 354-5355
Toll-free: 1-800-498-3610

Green Foods Corporation
320 North Graves Avenue
Oxnard, CA
USA
93030
Call for a distributor near you:
(805) 983-7470

Green Kamut Corporation
3397 E. 19th Street
Long Beach, CA
USA
90804
Call for a distributor near you:
(562) 498-5769

Greens+ Canada
94-689 Queen Street W.
Toronto, ON
Canada
M6J 1E6
Tel: (416) 977-3070
Fax: (416) 977-4184

Orange Peel Enterprises Inc.
2183 Ponce de Leon Circle
Vero Beach, FL
USA
32960
Tel: (561) 562-2766
Toll-free: 1-800-643-1210

Health Way Products
11 Sims Crescent, Unit 7
Richmond Hill, ON
Canada
L4B 1C9
Tel: (905) 731-8097
Fax: (905) 731-8116

K.R.P. Enterprises
5425 Beeler Avenue
Woodland Hills, CA
USA
91367
Tel: (818) 347-0387
Fax: (818) 594-0466

Herbon Naturals, Inc.
Unit 120-11300 River Road
Richmond, BC
Canada
V6X 1Z5
Tel: (604) 214-0705
Fax: (604) 214-0715

Holistic Horizons
338 N. Canal Street
Suite 22
South San Francisco, CA
USA
94080
Tel:(415) 871-8603
Fax: (415) 871-8606

Inno-Vite Inc.
196 Wildcat Road
Downsview, ON
Canada
M3J 2N5
Tel: (416) 661-8272
Fax: (416) 661-5992

Inno-Vite Inc.
196 Wildcat Road
Downsview, ON
Canada
M3J 2N5
Tel: (416) 661-8272
Fax: (416) 661-5992

Inter-Cal Corporation
533 Madison Avenue
Prescott, AZ
USA
86301
Tel: (520) 445-8063
Fax: (520) 778-7986

Kare & Hope Inc.
202-2345 Stanfield Road
Mississauga, ON
Canada
L4Y 3Y3
Tel:(905) 275-7546
Fax: (905) 275-8865

Klaire Laboratories, Inc. USA & Europe
1573 W. Seminole Street
San Marcos, CA
USA
92069
Tel: (619) 744-9680
Fax: (619) 744-9364

Klaire Laboratories
#19-7500 Cumberland Street
Burnaby, BC
Canada
V3N 4Z9
Tel: (604) 525-0868
Fax: (604) 521-2715
Toll-free: 1-888-913-4567

Vital Cell Life
Kanaalweg 17G
KL Utrecht
The Netherlands
3526
Tel: ++31-(0) 302-871008
Fax: ++31-(0) 302-871056

Bio-Mineral
Frauenstr 17
Muenchen 5
Germany
8000
Tel: ++49 89-225630
Fax: ++49 89-2289300

Health Interlink Ltd.
Interlink House
1A Crown Street
Redbaum, Hertfordshire
England
AL3 7JX
Tel: ++44 1582-794094
Fax: ++44 1582-794909

New Hope Nutrition Ltd.
P.O. Box 331147
Takauna, Auckland
New Zealand
9
Tel: ++64 9-489-4485
Fax: ++64 9-489-6515

Kyolic Ltd.
23501 Madero
Mission Viejo, CA
USA
92891
Tel: (714) 855-2776
Fax: (714) 458-2764

Quest Vitamins (BICL)
5180 South Service Road
Burlington, ON
Canada
L7L 5H4
Tel: (905) 637-7800
Fax: (905) 639-5293
Toll-free: 1-800-663-1412

Lane Labs USA Inc.
110 Commerce Drive
Allendale, NJ
USA
07401

Purity Life Health Products Ltd.
6 Commerce Crescent
Acton, ON
Canada
L7J 2X2
Tel: (519) 853-3511
Fax: (519) 853-4660
Toll-free: 1-800-265-2615

Lavilin™ Cosmetics
Hataasia Street, Industrial Zone
P.O. Box 444
Raanana
Israel
43661

Purity Life Health Products Ltd.
6 Commerce Crescent
Acton, ON
Canada
L7J 2X2
Tel: (519) 853-3511
Fax: (519) 853-4660
Toll-free: 1-800-265-2615

Life-Time Nutrition Inc.
Unit #107
12414-82nd Avenue
Surrey, BC
Canada
V3W 3E9
Tel: (604) 597-8050
Fax: (604) 597-6968

McZand® Herbal Inc.
P.O. Box 5312
Santa Monica, CA
USA
90409
Tel: (303) 786-8558
Fax: (303) 786-9435

Christmas Natural Foods
#203-8173 128th Street
Surrey, BC
Canada
V3W 4G1
Tel: (604) 591-8881
Fax: (604) 597-1784
Toll-free: 1-800-663-6559

Donmar Health & Beauty
259 Steelcase Road W.
Markham, ON
Canada
L3R 2P6
Tel: (905) 475-6530
Fax: (905) 475-9698
Toll-free: 1-800-757-4531

Purity Life Health Products Ltd.
6 Commerce Street
Acton, ON
Canada
L7J 2X3
Tel: (519) 853-3511
Fax: (519) 853-4660
Toll-free: 1-800-265-2615

Melbrosin International
Austria

Flora Manufacturing and Distributing Ltd.
7400 Fraser Park Drive
Burnaby, BC
Canada
V5J 5B9
Tel: (604) 436-6000
Fax: (604) 436-6060

naka Sales Ltd.
53 Queens Plate Drive, #3
Etobicoke, ON
Canada
M9W 6P1
Tel:(416) 748-3073
Fax: (416) 748-1555

naka Sales Ltd.
2221 Kenmore Avenue, #104
Buffalo, NY
USA
14207
Tel: (716) 447-1886
Fax: (716) 447-1884

Natren™ Inc.
3105 Willow Lane
Westlake Village, CA
USA
91361
Tel: (805) 371-4737
Fax: (805) 371-4742

Integrative Formulations
301-958 W. 8th Avenue
Vancouver, BC
Canada
V5Z 1E5
Tel: (604) 816-6245
Fax: (604) 732-9332

Cornucopia
260 Lake Road
Dayville, CT
USA
06241
Tel: (860) 779-2807
Fax: (203) 779-2811

Nature's Best
105 S. Puente Avenue
Brea, CA
USA
92621
Tel: (714) 441-2378
Fax: (714) 447-9218

Tree of Life (Midwest)
225 Daniels Way
Bloomington, IN
USA
47402
Tel: (812) 335-1511
Fax: (812) 335-6218

Tree of Life (Southeast)
4055 Deer Park Blvd
Elkton, FL
USA
32033
Tel: (904) 824-8181
Fax: (904) 825-2012

Natural Factors® Nutritional Products Ltd.
3655 Bonneville Place
Burnaby, BC
Canada
V3N 4S9
Tel: (604) 420-4229
Fax: (604) 420-0772

Natural Factors® Nutritional Products Ltd.
1420-80th Street S.W.
Suite B
Everett, WA
USA
98203
Tel: (425) 513-8800
Fax: (425) 348-9050
Toll-free: 1-800-322-8704

Nature's Herbs®
East 600 Quality Drive
American Fork, UT
USA
84003
Call for a distributor near you:
(801) 763-0700

Purity Life Health Products Ltd.
6 Commerce Crescent
Acton, ON
Canada
L7J 2M4
Tel: (519) 853-3511
Fax: (519) 853-4660
Toll-free: 1-800-265-2615

NaturPharm Inc.
32–7751 Yonge Street
Thornhill, ON
Canada
L3T 3N1
Call for a distributor near you:
(905) 764-2873

New Era® Natural Products Inc.
1491 South Miami Avenue
Miami, FL
USA
33130

Purity Life Health Products Ltd.
6 Commerce Crescent
Acton, ON
Canada
L7J 2X2
Tel: (519) 853-3511
Fax: (519) 853-4660
Toll-free: 1-800-265-2615

New Nordic
Denmark

Flora Manufacturing and Distributing Ltd.
7400 Fraser Park Drive
Burnaby, BC
Canada
V5J 5B9
Tel: (604) 436-6000
Fax: (604) 436-6060

Next Nutrition
P.O. Box 2469
Carlsbad, CA
USA
92018
Tel: (760) 431-8152
Fax: (760) 431-9969

Upper 49th Imports
1463 Dugald Road
Winnipeg, MB
Canada
R2J 0H3
Tel: (204) 233-3132
Fax: (204) 237-7019
Toll-free: 1-800-563-0965

Nova® Homeopathic Therapeutics Inc.
5600 McLeod N.E., Suite F
Albuquerque, NM
USA
87109
Call for a distributor near you:
(505) 883-5672

Purity Life Health Products Ltd.
6 Commerce Crescent
Acton, ON
Canada
L7J 2X2
Tel: (519) 853-3511
Fax: (519) 853-4660
Toll-free: 1-800-265-2615

Palko Distributing Co., Inc.
792 McCool Road
Valparaiso, IN
USA
46383
Fax: 1-888-759-1199
Toll-free: 1-800-759-4931

Super-Nutrition Distributors, Inc.
P.O. Box 2383947
Austin Boulevard
Island Park, NY
USA
11558-1248
Tel: (516) 897-2480
Fax: (516) 897-2580

Tucson Cooperative
Warehouse
350 S. Toole Avenue
Tucson, AZ
USA
85701
Tel: (520) 884-9951
Fax: (520) 792-3241

Novartis Nutrition Inc.
Gran Via De La Corts
Catalanes, Barcelona
Spain
76408013
Tel: 41 31 377-6154
Fax: 41 31 377-6944

Inno-Vite Inc.
196 Wildcat Road
Downsview, ON
Canada
M3J 2N5
Tel: (416) 661-8272
Fax: (416) 661-5992

Nu-Life Nutrition Ltd.™
8920 Woodbine Avenue
Markham, ON
Canada
L3R 9W9
Tel: (905) 475-3500
Fax: (905) 475-3355

Nu-Life Nutrition Ltd.™
150-13160 Vanier Place
Richmond, BC
Canada
V6V 2J2
Tel: (604) 273-8366
Fax: (604) 278-3679
Toll-free: 1-888-868-5433
Western Office

Nu-Life Nutrition Ltd.™
55 Boul. Montpellier
St. Laurent, QC
Canada
H4N 2G3
Tel: (514) 744-4200
Fax: (514) 744-4202
Toll-free: 1-800-667-2354

Nutra Research
International
7411 McCallan Road
Richmond, BC
Canada
V7C 2H6
Tel: (604) 274-6116
Fax: (604) 274-6119

Nutraceutics Corporation
105-600 Fairway Drive
Deerfield Beach, FL
USA
33441
Tel: (954) 725-3000
Fax: (954) 725-3904

Nutrex® Inc.
73-4460 Queen Kaahumanu
Hwy., #102
Kailua-Kona, HI
USA
96740
Call for a distributor near you:
(808) 329-4677

Nutribiotic
(Bio-Chem Research)
865 Parallel Drive
Lakeport, CA
USA
95453
Tel: (707) 263-1475
Fax: (707) 263-7844

Ecotrend Products Ltd.
202-188 West 6th Avenue
Vancouver, BC
Canada
V5Y 1K6
Tel: (604) 876-9876
Fax: (604) 876-9846

Padma
CH-8702
Zollikon
Switzerland
Tel:++41 1 391-9555
Fax: ++41 1 391-9818

Inno-Vite Inc.
196 Wildcat Road
Downsview, ON
Canada
M3J 2N5
Tel: (416) 661-8272
Fax: (416) 661-5992

Pharmaton
900 Ridgebury Road
P.O. Box 368
Ridgefield, CT
USA
06877
Tel: (203) 798-4628
Fax: (203) 798-5771

Quest Vitamins
5180 South Service Road
Burlington, ON
Canada
L7L 5H4
Tel: (905) 637-7800
Fax: (905) 639-5293

Power Health Products Ltd.
Airfield Estate
Pocklington, Yorkshire
England
Y04 2NR
Tel:++44 1759 304551
Fax: ++44 1759 304551

Inno-Vite Inc.
196 Wildcat Road
Downsview, ON
Canada
M3J 2N5
Tel: (416) 661-8272
Fax: (416) 661-5992

Prairie Naturals®
Unit 108B
1772 Broadway Street
Port Coquitlam, BC
Canada
V3C 2M8
Tel: (604) 941-4950
Fax: (604) 941-4974

Corwin Distribution
195 Signet Drive
North York, ON
Canada
M9L 1V1
Tel: (416) 747-1942
Fax: (416) 747-1479
Toll-free: 1-800-464-5116

Pure-Gar®
10029 South Tacoma Way
Suite E-6
Tacoma, WA
USA
98499
Tel: (253) 582-6421
Fax: (253) 582-6734

Pure Source
Highway 24 South RR #7
Guelph, ON
Canada
N1H 6J4
Tel: (519) 837-2140

Donmar Health Foods
259 Steelcase Road West
Markham, ON
Canada
L3R 2P6
Tel: (905) 475-6530

Christmas Natural Foods
#203-8173 128th Street
Surrey, BC
Canada
V3W 4G1
Tel: (604) 591-8881

Star Marketing
19720-94A Avenue, Unit D
Suite 107
Langley, BC
Canada
V1M 2B7
Tel: (604) 888-4049

Cornucopia Natural Foods
260 Lake Road
Dayville, CT
USA
06241
Tel: (203) 779-2800

Food For Health
3655 West Washington
Phoenix, AZ
USA
85005
Tel: (602) 269-2371

Mountain People's
Warehouse
4005 Sixth Avenue South
Seattle, WA
USA
981108
Tel: (206) 467-7190

Nature's Best
105 South Puente Street
Brea, CA
USA
92621
Tel: (714) 441-2378

Rainbow Natural Foods
4850 Moline Street
Denver, CO
USA
80239
Tel: (303) 373-1144

Stow Mills
71 Stow Drive
Chesterfield, NH
USA
03443
Tel: (603) 256-3000

Tree of Life Divisions
Toll-free: 1-800-874-0851

Quest Vitamins
5180 South Service Road
Burlington, ON
Canada
L7L 5H4
Tel:(905) 637-7800
Fax: (905) 639-5293

Salus-Haus
Bruckmühl/Mangfall Obb.
Germany
D-83052
Tel:++49 8062 9010
Fax: ++49 8062 9197

Flora Manufacturing and
Distributing Ltd.
7400 Fraser Park Drive
Burnaby, BC
Canada
V5J 5B9
Tel: (604) 436-6000
Fax: (604) 436-6060

Scandinavian Natural
Health & Beauty
Products, Inc.
13 N. 7th Street
Perkasie, PA
USA
18944
Call for a distributor near you:
(215) 453-2505

Sisu™ Enterprises Co. Inc.
104A-3430 Brighton Avenue
Burnaby, BC
Canada
V5A 3H4
Call for a distributor near you:
(604) 420-6610

Standard Homeopathic
and P&S Laboratories
210 W. 131st Street
Los Angeles, CA
USA
90061
Call for a distributor near you:
(213) 321-4284

Standard Homeopathic
Canada
P.O. Box 1019
Sutton, QC
Canada
J0E 2K0
Tel: (514) 522-4556
Fax: (514) 538-6638
Toll-free: 1-800-363-8933
Eastern Representatives

Standard Homeopathic
2347 Sumpter Drive
Coquitlam, BC
Canada
V3J 6Y3
Tel: (604) 461-5512
Fax: (604) 461-5512
Toll-free: 1-888-477-8899
Western Representatives

Sun Force International
P.O. Box 2549
Vancouver, BC
Canada
V6B 3W8
Call for a distributor near you:
(604) 532-0892

Synpharma
Switzerland

Flora Manufacturing and
Distributing Ltd.
7400 Fraser Park Drive
Burnaby, BC
Canada
V5J 5B9
Tel: (604) 436-6000
Fax: (604) 436-6060

The Green Turtle Bay®
Vitamin Co., Inc.
P.O. Box 642
56 High Street
Summit, NJ
USA
07901
Call for a distributor near you:
(908) 277-2240

The Real Aloe®
Company, Inc.
P.O. Box 2770
Oxnard, CA
USA
93033
Call for a distributor near you:
(805) 483-4408

J. Gahler International
205-20050 Stewart Crescent
Maple Ridge, BC
Canada
V2X 0T4
Tel: (604) 465-9595
Fax: (604) 465-0434

Swiss Herbal Remedies
Limited
35 Leek Crescent
Richmond Hill, ON
Canada
L4B 4C2
Tel: (905) 886-9500

UAS Labs
5610 Rowland Road
Unit 110
Minnetonka, MN
USA
55343
Fax: (612) 935-1650

Inno-Vite Inc.
196 Wildcat Road
Downsview, ON
Canada
M3J 2N5
Tel: (416) 661-8272
Fax: (416) 661-5992

Uncle Lee's Teas® Inc.
11020 Rush Street
South El Monte, CA
USA
91733
Tel: (626) 350-3309
Fax: (626) 350-4364

Koyo Foods Inc.
393 St. Croix, Suite A
Montreal, QC
Canada
Tel: (514) 744-1299
Fax: (514) 744-0882

Christmas Natural Foods
203-8173 128th Street
Surrey, BC
Canada
V3W 4G1
Tel: (604) 591-8881
Fax: (604) 597-1784

Nature's Best
105 S. Puente Street
Brea, CA
USA
92621
Tel: (714) 441-2378
Fax: (714) 441-2330

Cornucopia Natural
Foods, Inc.
260 Lake Road
Dayville, CT
USA
06241
Tel: (860) 779-2807
Fax: (860) 779-2811

Vita Health Co. Ltd.
150 Beghin Avenue
Winnipeg, MB
Canada
R2J 3W2
Tel: (204) 661-8386
Fax: (204) 663-8386

W. Schoenenberger
Germany

Flora Manufacturing and
Distributing Ltd.
7400 Fraser Park Drive
Burnaby, BC
Canada
V5J 5B9
Tel: (604) 436-6000
Fax: (604) 436-6060

Wakunaga of America
Co., Ltd.
23501 Madero
Mission Viego, CA
USA
92691-2764
Tel: (714) 855-2776
Fax: (714) 458-2764

Quest Vitamins (BICL)
5180 South Service Road
Burlington, ON
Canada
L7L 5H4
Tel: (905) 637-7800
Fax: (905) 639-3769
Toll-free: 1-800-663-1412

Wild Rose Laboratories
8173-128th Street, #201
Surrey, BC
Canada
V3W 4G1
Tel: (604) 591-8881
Fax: (604) 597-1784

Christmas Natural Foods
203-8173 128th Street
Surrey, BC
Canada
V3W 4G1
Tel: (604) 591-8881
Fax: (604) 597-1784
Toll-free: 1-800-663-6559
Western Canada

Yves Ponroy, Institut de
Recherche Biologique
78340 Les Clayes-sous-Bois
France
Tel: ++33 (1) 30 70 69 00
Fax: ++33 (1) 30 79 69 78

Yves Ponroy Canada Inc.
8568 Boul. PIE IX
Montreal, QC
Canada
H1Z 4G2
Tel: (514) 376-6990
Fax: (514) 376-3539

Visual
Identification

Section III

This section provides photographs of the product packaging for many of the products in the Product listing section to simplify identification at your local retailer. Those products included are in alphabetical order by product brand name.

Visual Identification

Products that have a "Visual Identification" symbol in the "Product Listings" section
are listed here. All photographs are in alphabetical order by product name.

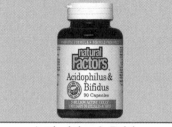

Acidophilus & Bifidus
Natural Factors® Nutritional Products Ltd.

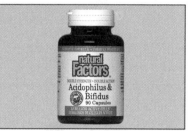

**Acidophilus & Bifidus
Double Strength**
Natural Factors® Nutritional Products Ltd.

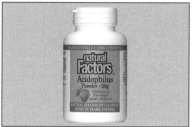

Acidophilus Powder
Natural Factors® Nutritional Products Ltd.

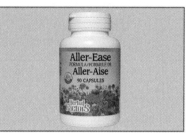

Aller-Ease Formula
Natural Factors® Nutritional Products Ltd.

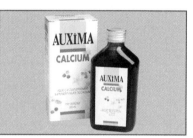

Auxima Calcium
Novartis Nutrition Inc.

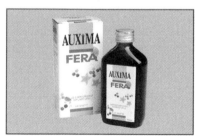

Auxima Fera
Novartis Nutrition Inc.

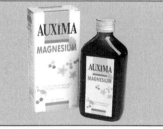

Auxima Magnesium
Novartis Nutrition Inc.

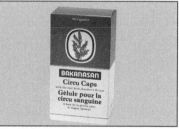

Bakanasan Circu-Caps™
Börner GmbH

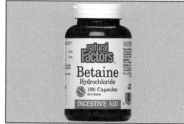

Betaine Hydrochloride
Natural Factor® Nutritional Products Ltd.

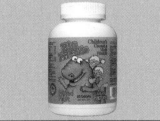

**Big Friends Children's
Chewable Multi Vitamin**
Natural Factors® Nutritional Products Ltd.

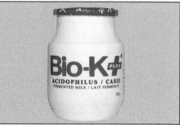

Bio-K Plus™
Bio-K+™ International Inc.

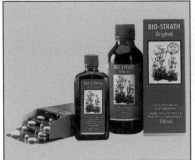

**Bio-Strath Herbal
Yeast Food Supplements**
Bio-Strath AG®

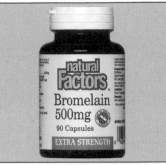

Bromelain 500 mg
Natural Factors® Nutritional Products Ltd.

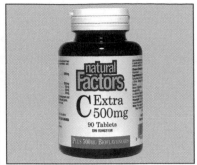

C Extra 500 mg
Natural Factors® Nutritional Products Ltd.

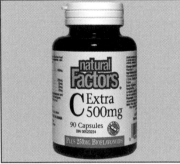

C Extra 500 mg
Natural Factors® Nutritional Products Ltd.

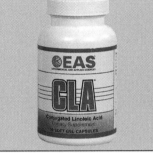

CLA™ (U.S.)
EAS

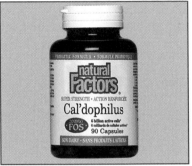

Cal'dophilus Super Strength
Natural Factors® Nutritional Products Ltd.

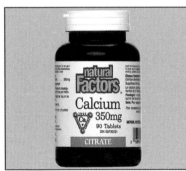

Calcium 350 mg
Natural Factors® Nutritional Products Ltd.

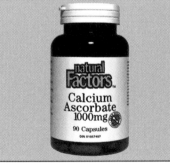

Calcium Ascorbate 1000 mg
Natural Factors® Nutritional Products Ltd.

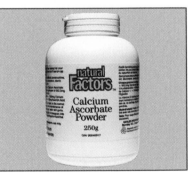

Calcium Ascorbate Powder
Natural Factors® Nutritional Products Ltd.

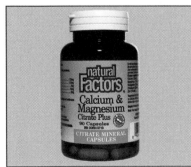

**Calcium & Magnesium
Citrate Plus**
Natural Factors® Nutritional Products Ltd.

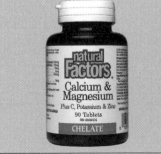

**Calcium & Magnesium
Plus C, Potassium & Zinc**
Natural Factors® Nutritional Products Ltd.

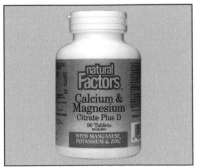

**Calcium & Magnesium
Citrate Plus D**
Natural Factors® Nutritional Products Ltd.

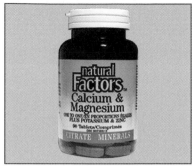

**Calcium & Magnesium
Citrate Plus Potassium & Zinc**
Natural Factors® Nutritional Products Ltd.

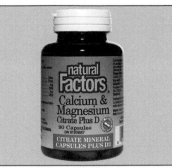

**Calcium & Magnesium
Citrate Plus D3**
Natural Factors® Nutritional Products Ltd.

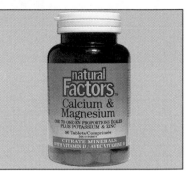

**Calcium & Magnesium
Citrate Plus D**
Natural Factors® Nutritional Products Ltd.

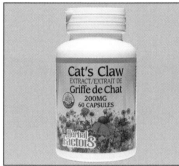

Cat's Claw Extract
Natural Factors® Nutritional Products Ltd.

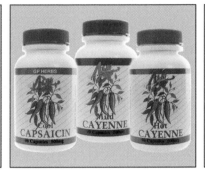

Cayenne
Albi Imports Ltd.

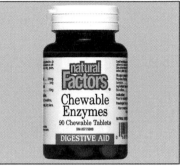

Chewable Enzymes
Natural Factors® Nutritional Products Ltd.

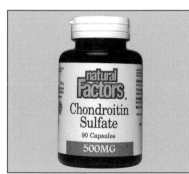

Chondroitin Sulfate
Natural Factors® Nutritional Products Ltd.

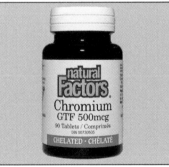

Chromium GTF 500 mcg
Natural Factors® Nutritional Products Ltd.

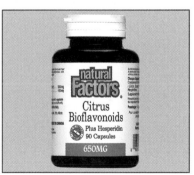

Citrus Bioflavonoids
Natural Factors® Nutritional Products Ltd.

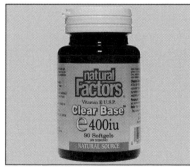

Clear Base™ E 400 iu
Natural Factors® Nutritional Products Ltd.

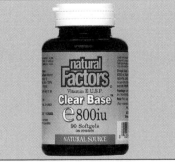

Clear Base™ E 800 iu
Natural Factors® Nutritional Products Ltd.

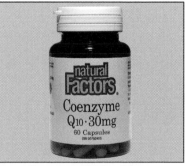

Coenzyme Q10 • 30 mg
Natural Factors® Nutritional Products Ltd.

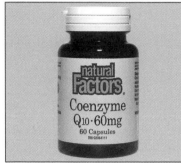

Coenzyme Q10 • 60 mg
Natural Factors® Nutritional Products Ltd.

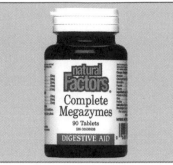

Complete Megazymes
Natural Factors® Nutritional Products Ltd.

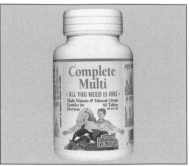

Complete Multi
Natural Factors® Nutritional Products Ltd.

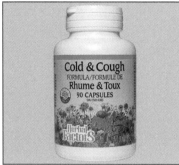

Cough & Cold Formula
Natural Factors® Nutritional Products Ltd.

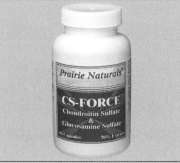

CS-Force™ Chondroitin Sulfate
Prairie Naturals®

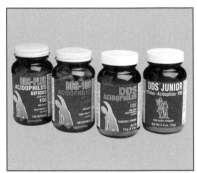

DDS Acidophilus®
UAS Labs

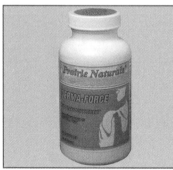

Derma-Force™
Prairie Naturals®

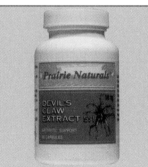

Devil's Claw Extract 5:1
Prairie Naturals®

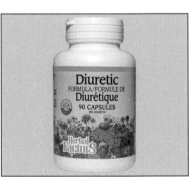

Diuretic Formula
Natural Factors® Nutritional Products Ltd.

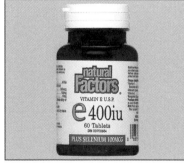

E 400 iu Plus Selenium 100 mcg
Natural Factors® Nutritional Products Ltd.

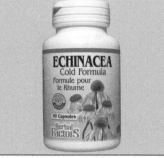

Echinacea Cold Formula
Natural Factors® Nutritional Products Ltd.

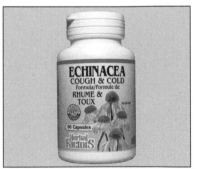

Echinacea Cough & Cold Formula
Natural Factors® Nutritional Products Ltd.

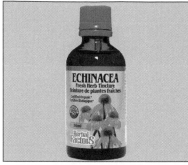

Echinacea Fresh Herb Tincture
Natural Factors® Nutritional Products Ltd.

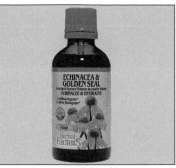

Echinacea & Goldenseal
Natural Factors® Nutritional Products Ltd.

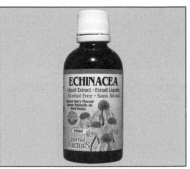

Echinacea Liquid Extract
Natural Factors® Nutritional Products Ltd.

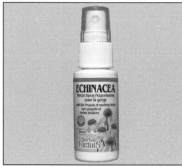

Echinacea Throat Spray
Natural Factors® Nutritional Products Ltd.

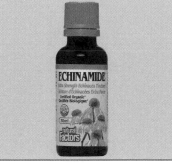

Echinacea Tincture
Natural Factors® Nutritional Products Ltd.

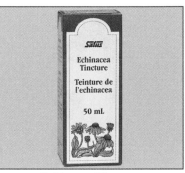

Echinacea Tincture
Salus-Haus

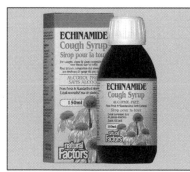

Echinamide™ Cough Syrup
Natural Factors® Nutritional Products Ltd.

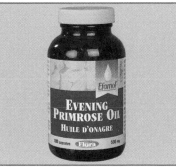

Efamol® Evening Primrose Oil
Efamol Research Institute

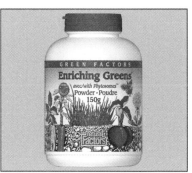

Enriching Greens®
Natural Factors® Nutritional Products Ltd.

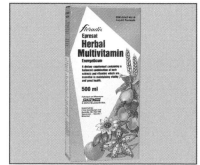

Epresat Herbal Multivitamin
Salus-Haus

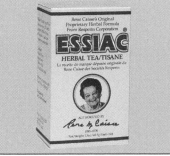

Essiac® Herbal Formula
Essiac® International

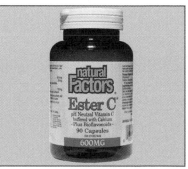

Ester C® 600 mg
Plus Bioflavonoids
Natural Factors® Nutritional Products Ltd.

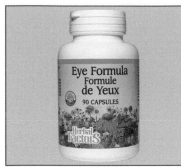

Eye Formula
Natural Factors® Nutritional Products Ltd.

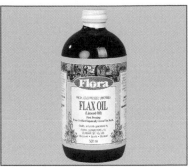

Flax Oil
Flora Manufacturing & Distributing Ltd.

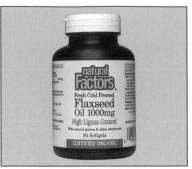

Flaxseed Oil 1000 mg
Natural Factors® Nutritional Products Ltd.

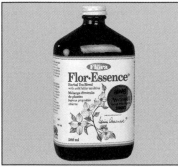

Flor-Essence Herbal Tea Blend®
Flora Manufacturing & Distributing Ltd.

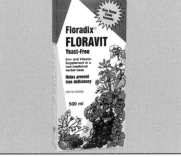

Floradix® Floravit
Salus-Haus

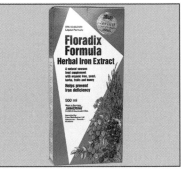

Floradix® Formula
Salus-Haus

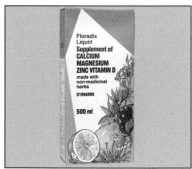

**Floradix® Liquid Calcium
Magnesium-Zinc and Vitamin D**
Salus-Haus

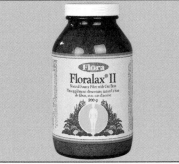

FloraLax® II
Flora Manufacturing & Distributing Ltd.

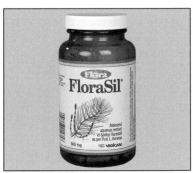

FloraSil® (formerly "VegeSil")
Flora Manufacturing & Distributing Ltd.

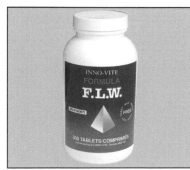

Formula F. L. W.®
Inno-Vite Inc.

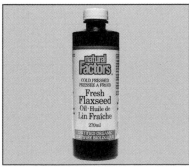

Fresh Cold Pressed Flaxseed Oil
Natural Factors® Nutritional Products Ltd.

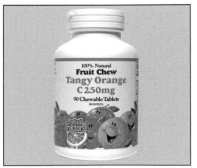

**Fruit Chew Tangy Orange
C 250 mg**
Natural Factors® Nutritional Products Ltd.

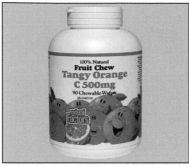

**Fruit Chew Tangy Orange
C 500 mg**
Natural Factors® Nutritional Products Ltd.

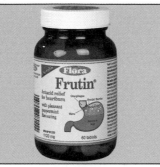

Frutin®
New Nordic

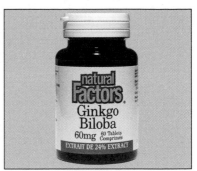

Ginkgo Biloba
Natural Factors® Nutritional Products Ltd.

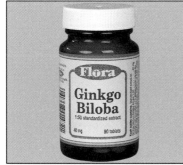

Ginkgo Biloba
Flora Manufacturing & Distributing Ltd.

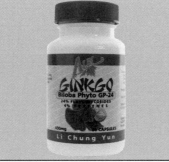

Ginkgo Biloba Phyto GP-24
Albi Imports Ltd.

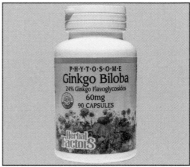

Ginkgo Biloba Phytosome™
Natural Factors® Nutritional Products Ltd.

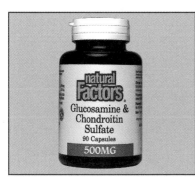

**Glucosamine &
Chondroitin Sulfate**
Natural Factors® Nutritional Products Ltd.

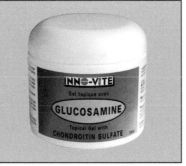

Glucosamine Topical Gel
Inno-Vite Inc.

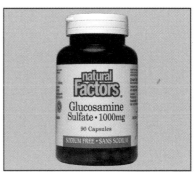

Glucosamine Sulfate 1000 mg
Natural Factors® Nutritional Products Ltd.

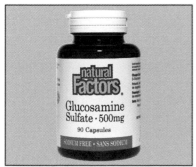

Glucosamine Sulfate 500 mg
Natural Factors® Nutritional Products Ltd.

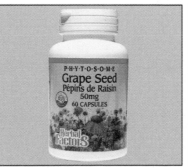

Grape Seed Phytosome™
Natural Factors® Nutritional Products Ltd.

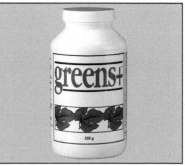

Greens+™
Greens+™ Canada

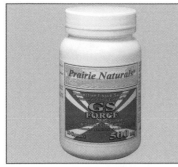

GS Force™
Prairie Naturals®

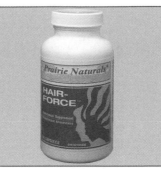

Hair-Force™
Prairie Naturals®

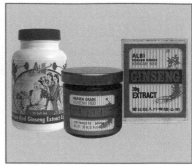

Heaven Grade Korean Red Ginseng
Albi Imports Ltd.

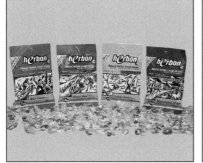

**Herbon™ Adventurous Tingle™
Herbal Cough Drops**
Herbon Naturals, Inc.

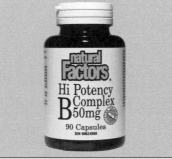

Hi Potency B Complex
Natural Factors® Nutritional Products Ltd.

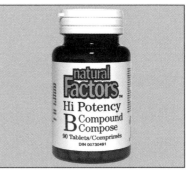

Hi Potency B Compound
Natural Factors® Nutritional Products Ltd.

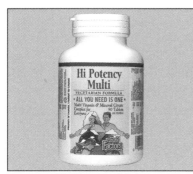

Hi Potency Multi
Natural Factors® Nutritional Products Ltd.

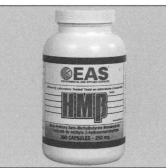

HMB™ (U.S.)
EAS

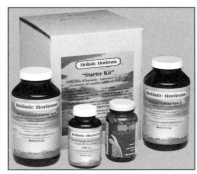

Holistic Horizon's Starter Kit®
Holistic Horizons

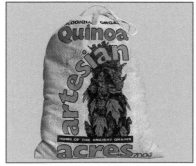

Inca-Rice™ Golden Quinoa
Artesian Acres Inc.

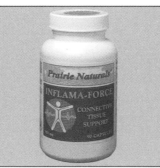

Inflama-Force
Prairie Naturals®

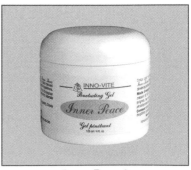

Inner Peace®
Inno-Vite Inc.

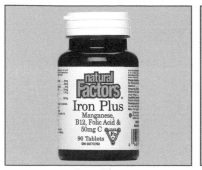

Iron Plus
Natural Factors® Nutritional Products Ltd.

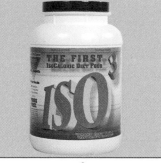

ISO³®
Next Nutrition

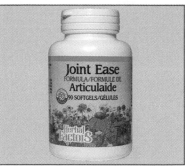

Joint Ease Formula
Natural Factors® Nutritional Products Ltd.

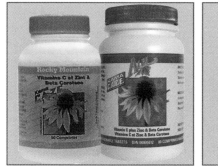

KAMA C.A.Z.E.
Albi Imports Ltd.

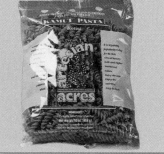

Kamut®
Artesian Acres Inc.

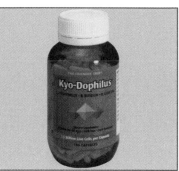

Kyo-Dophilus®
Wakunaga of America Co., Ltd.

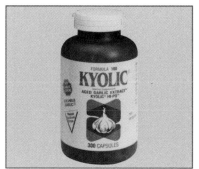

Kyolic® Aged Garlic Extract™
Wakunaga of America Co., Ltd.

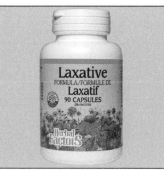

Laxative Formula
Natural Factors® Nutritional Products Ltd.

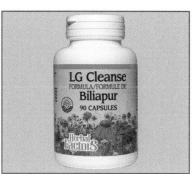

LG Cleanse Formula
Natural Factors® Nutritional Products Ltd.

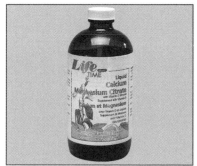

Liquid Calcium-Magnesium Citrate
Life-Time Nutrition Inc.

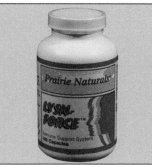

Lysn-Force™
Prairie Naturals®

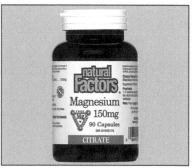

Magnesium Citrate
Natural Factors® Nutritional Products Ltd.

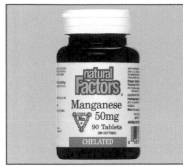

Manganese Chelated
Natural Factors® Nutritional Products Ltd.

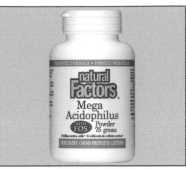

Mega Acidophilus Powder with FOS
Natural Factors® Nutritional Products Ltd.

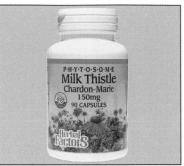

Milk Thistle Phytosome™
Natural Factors® Nutritional Products Ltd.

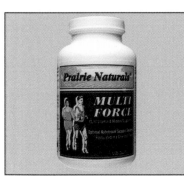

Milk Thistle Tonic
Anton Huebner GmbH & CO KG

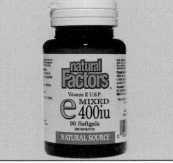

Mixed E 400 iu
Natural Factors® Nutritional Products Ltd.

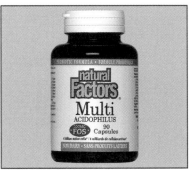

Multi Acidophilus
Natural Factors® Nutritional Products Ltd.

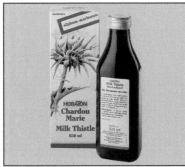

Multi-Force™
Prairie Naturals®

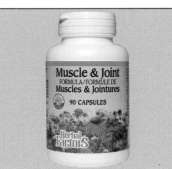

Muscle & Joint Formula
Natural Factors® Nutritional Products Ltd.

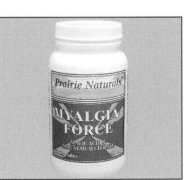

Myalgia-Force™
Prairie Naturals®

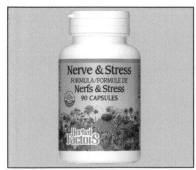

Nerve & Stress Formula
Natural Factors® Nutritional Products Ltd.

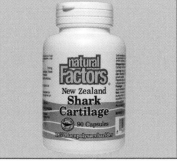

New Zealand Shark Cartilage
Natural Factors® Nutritional Products Ltd.

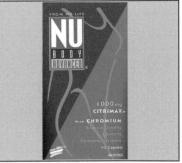

Nu-Body Advanced® 1000 mg Citrimax™
Nu-Life Nutrition Ltd.™

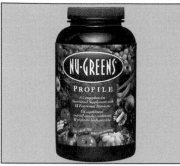

Nu-Greens® Profile
Nu-Life Nutrition Ltd.™

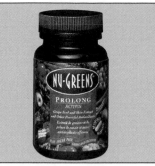

Nu-Greens® Prolong
Nu-Life Nutrition Ltd.™

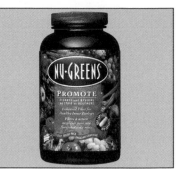

Nu-Greens® Promote
Nu-Life Nutrition Ltd.™

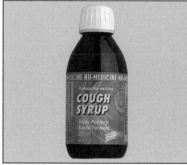

Nu-Medicine® Cough Syrup
Nu-Life Nutrition Ltd.™

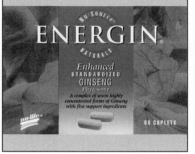

Nu-Source® Energin®
Nu-Life Nutrition Ltd.™

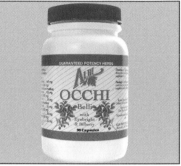

Occhi Belli
Albi Imports Ltd.

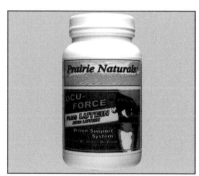

Ocu-Force™
Prairie Naturals®

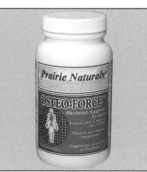

Osteo-Force™
Prairie Naturals®

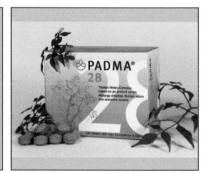

Padma 28®
Padma

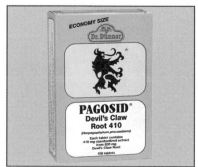

Pagosid™ Devil's Claw Root 410
Dr. Dunner AG

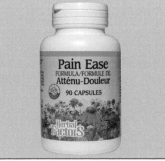

Pain Ease Formula
Natural Factors® Nutritional Products Ltd.

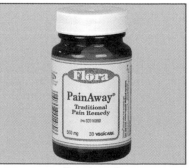

PainAway®
Flora Manufacturing & Distributing Ltd.

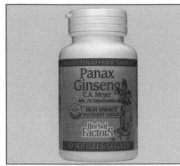

Panax Ginseng C.A. Meyer
Natural Factors® Nutritional Products Ltd.

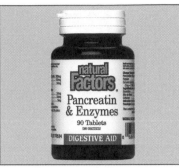

Pancreatin & Enzymes
Natural Factors® Nutritional Products Ltd.

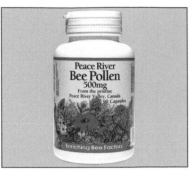

Peace River Bee Pollen 500 mg
Natural Factors® Nutritional Products Ltd.

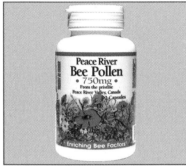

Peace River Bee Pollen 750 mg
Natural Factors® Nutritional Products Ltd.

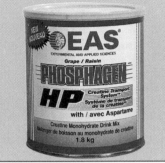

Phosphagen HP™ (U.S.)
EAS

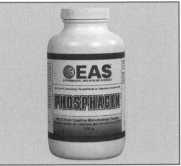

Phosphagen™ (U.S.)
EAS

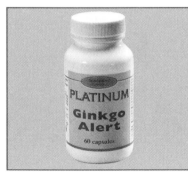

Platinum Ginkgo Alert
Health Way Products

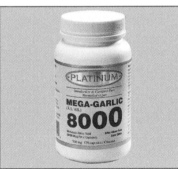

Platinum Mega-Garlic 8000
Health Way Products

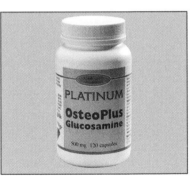

Platinum Osteo Plus Glucosamine
Health Way Products

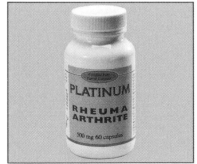

Platinum Rheuma Arthrite
Health Way Products

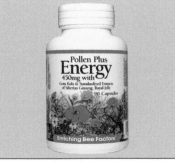

Pollen Plus Energy
Natural Factors® Nutritional Products Ltd.

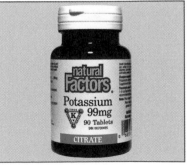

Potassium Citrate
Natural Factors® Nutritional Products Ltd.

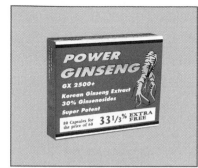

Power Ginseng GX 2500+
Power Health Products Ltd.

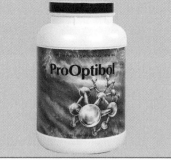

ProOptibol®
Next Nutrition

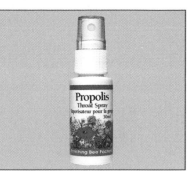

Propolis Throat Spray
Natural Factors® Nutritional Products Ltd.

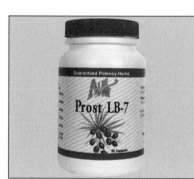

Propolis Tincture Extract 65%
Natural Factors® Nutritional Products Ltd.

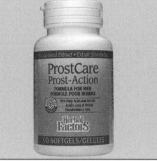

ProstCare Prost-Action
Natural Factors® Nutritional Products Ltd.

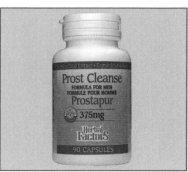

Prost Cleanse Formula For Men
Natural Factors® Nutritional Products Ltd.

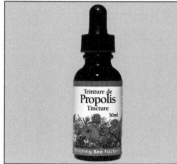

Prost LB-7
Albi Imports Ltd.

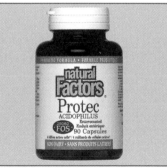

Protec Acidophilus
Natural Factors® Nutritional Products Ltd.

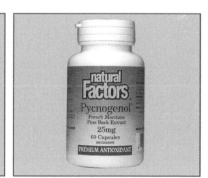

**Pycnogenol® French Maritime
Pine Bark Extract**
Natural Factors® Nutritional Products Ltd.

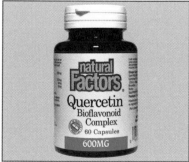

Quercetin Bioflavonoid Complex
Natural Factors® Nutritional Products Ltd.

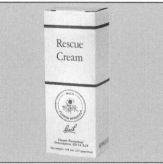

Rescue Cream
Bach Flower Remedies® Ltd.

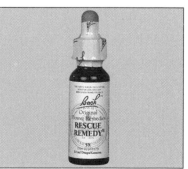

Rescue Remedy
Bach Flower Remedies® Ltd.

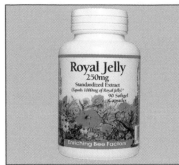

Royal Jelly 250 mg
Natural Factors® Nutritional Products Ltd.

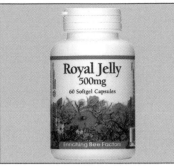

Royal Jelly 500 mg
Natural Factors® Nutritional Products Ltd.

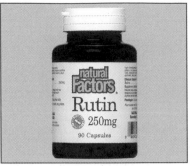

Rutin 250 mg
Natural Factors® Nutritional Products Ltd.

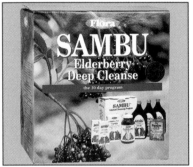

Sambu® Elderberry Deep Cleanse
Flora Manufacturing & Distributing Ltd.

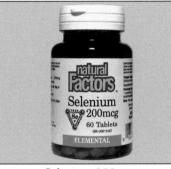

Selenium 200 mcg
Natural Factors® Nutritional Products Ltd.

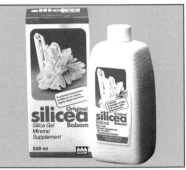

Silicea Gel
Anton Huebner GmbH & CO KG

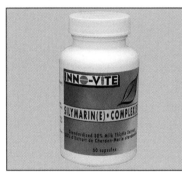

Silymarin Complex
Inno-Vite Inc.

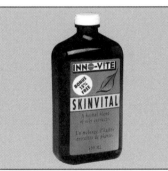

SKINVITAL®
Inno-Vite Inc.

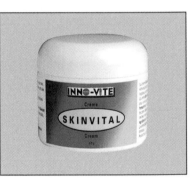

SKINVITAL® Cream
Inno-Vite Inc.

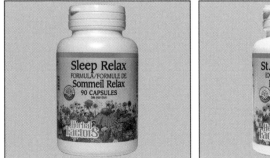

Sleep Relax Formula
Natural Factors® Nutritional Products Ltd.

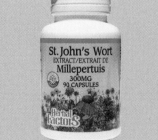

St. John's Wort Extract
Natural Factors® Nutritional Products Ltd.

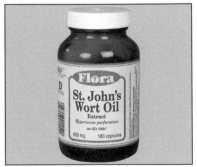

St. John's Wort Oil Extract
Flora Manufacturing & Distributing Ltd.

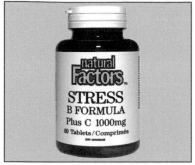

Stress B Formula Plus C 1000 mg
Natural Factors® Nutritional Products Ltd.

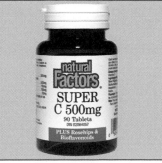

Super C 500 mg
Natural Factors® Nutritional Products Ltd.

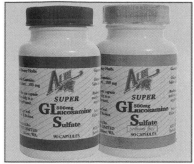

Super Glucosamine Sulfate
Albi Imports Ltd.

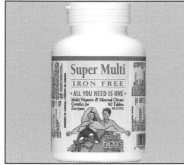

Super Multi
Natural Factors® Nutritional Products Ltd.

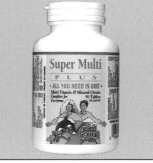

Super Multi Plus
Natural Factors® Nutritional Products Ltd.

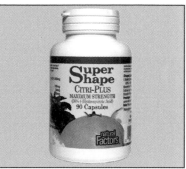

Super Shape Citri-Plus
Natural Factors® Nutritional Products Ltd.

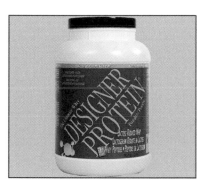

**The Ultimate Whey
Designer Protein®**
Next Nutrition

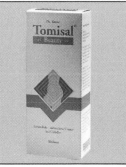

Tomisal™
Biolinea GmbH

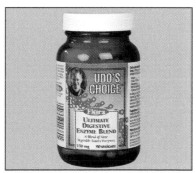

**Udo's Choice® Ultimate Digestive
Enzyme Blend**
Flora Manufacturing & Distributing Ltd.

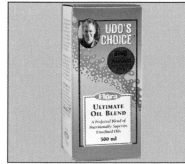

**Udo's Choice® Ultimate
Oil Blend®**
Flora Manufacturing & Distributing Ltd.

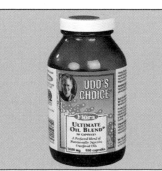

**Udo's Choice® Ultimate
Oil Blend® Capsules**
Flora Manufacturing & Distributing Ltd.

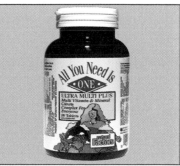

Ultra Multi Plus
Natural Factors® Nutritional Products Ltd.

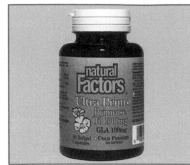

Ultra Prim Primrose Oil 1000 mg
Natural Factors® Nutritional Products Ltd.

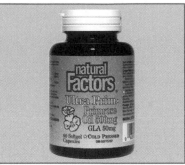

Ultra Prim Primrose Oil 500 mg
Natural Factors® Nutritional Products Ltd.

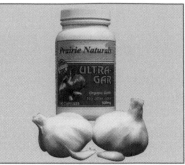

Ultra-Gar™
Prairie Naturals®

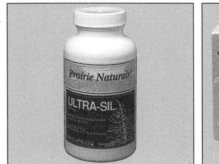

Ultra-Sil
Prairie Naturals®

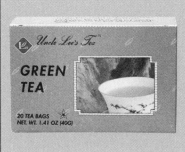

Uncle Lee's Green Teas®
Uncle Lee's Teas® Inc.

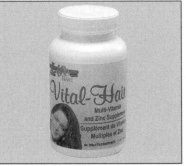

**Vital-Hair Multi-Vitamin
Supplement**
Life-Time Nutrition Inc.

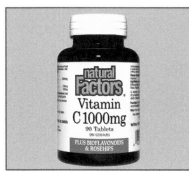

**Vitamin C 1000 mg Plus
Bioflavonoids & Rosehips**
Natural Factors® Nutritional Products Ltd.

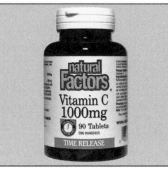

**Vitamin C 1000 mg
Time Release**
Natural Factors® Nutritional Products Ltd.

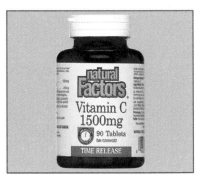

**Vitamin C 1500 mg
Time Release**
Natural Factors® Nutritional Products Ltd.

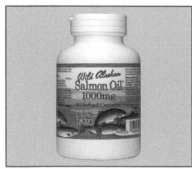

Wild Alaskan Salmon Oil 1000 mg
Natural Factors® Nutritional Products Ltd.

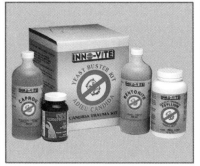

Yeast Buster Kit
Inno-Vite Inc.

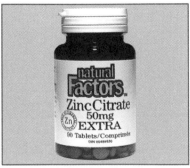

Zinc Citrate
Natural Factors® Nutritional Products Ltd.